Torah in a Time of Plague

Historical and Contemporary Jewish Responses

Edited by
Erin Leib Smokler

Ben Yehuda Press
Teaneck, New Jersey

Published by Ben Yehuda Press
122 Ayers Court #1B
Teaneck, NJ 07666

http://www.BenYehudaPress.com

To subscribe to our monthly book club and support independent Jewish publishing, visit https://www.patreon.com/BenYehudaPress

Ben Yehuda Press books may be purchased at a discount by synagogues, book clubs, and other institutions buying in bulk. For information, please email markets@BenYehudaPress.com

Cover image from the 'Golden Haggadah', c. 1320-1330, Catalonia, Spain. British Library MS 27210.

Grateful acknowledgement is made to the original publishers of the following essays, for permitting their reprint in this volume:

Tamara Mann Tweel, "The Song of Sirens: Giving Birth at the Height of the Pandemic," Tablet Magazine, December 11, 2020.

Shaul Magid, "COVID 19 and the Theological Challenge of the Arbitrary," Jewish Social Studies, Fall 2020, Vol. 26, No. 1, pp. 33-45.

ISBN13 978-1-953829-09-2

21 22 23 / 10 9 8 7 6 5 4 3 2 1   20210430

Contents

Introduction:
Theological Vertigo in Proximity to Plague

Erin Leib Smokler

The year 2020 has been marked by loss. Loss of life. Loss of jobs. Loss of community. Loss of physical and mental wellbeing. Loss of stability and predictability. Beyond the bodily pains wrought by illness, existential and spiritual struggles have challenged our centeredness. Loss tends to violate our senses of who we are in the world or the solidity of the world itself. It often lifts the veil on our own blind spots and compromises the plausibility structures that hold our lives intact. The Covid-19 pandemic has pressed us in all of these ways, demanding that those who survive live with death regularly, or at least in proximity to it. The consequences are weighty.

The Bible attests to the weightiness of this proximity through the story of Sarah's death.

> (1) And the life of Sarah was one hundred years and twenty years and seven years; [these were] the years of the life of Sarah. (2) And Sarah died in Kiriat Arba, which is Hebron, in the land of Canaan, and Abraham came to eulogize Sarah and to weep for her. (Genesis 23)

The life of Sarah (*hayey Sarah*) is characterized by her death, which famously follows the near-death of her son Isaac in the verses prior. The medieval commentator Rashi (1040-1105) explains this juxtaposition thus:

> "To eulogize Sarah and to weep for her": The account of Sarah's demise was juxtaposed to the binding of Isaac because as a result of the news of the "binding," that her son was prepared for slaughter and was almost slaughtered (*kimat she'lo nishchat*), her soul flew out of her, and she died. (Rashi on 23:2)

On the one hand, one could say that Isaac's ordeal broke his mother's heart and caused it to shatter. But that phrase "*kimat she'lo nishchat*" is arresting. Isaac did not die and she knew it, according to Rashi. What, then,

1

was the cause of her death?

R. Judah Loew b. Bezalel (1520-1609), known as the Maharal of Prague, suggests the following:

> "And was almost slaughtered" (Rashi)... It seems that because [Sarah] heard that [Isaac] was almost slaughtered—that just a small thing [*davar muat*] kept him from being slaughtered—for this reason she was shocked [*nivhala*]. This is the way of humanity: to be shocked upon hearing that only a small thing kept one alive. (*Gur Aryeh al ha-Torah, Hayey Sarah*)

It was the proximity of her son to death that shook Sarah to her core. The fact that a mere moment, "just a small thing," separated him from a fatal fate undid her. The seeming unpredictability of it all, the ease with which the story could have ended differently, rattled Sarah beyond reconstitution.

The contemporary biblical commentator Avivah Zornberg reads this poignantly, focusing her attention on the word "*nivhal.*"

> What is *behala*? Again, one could say something like shock. But *nivhal* is not exactly shock. *Nivhal* is something like dizziness, even a kind of nausea. It's vertigo. It's not knowing where one is, a shock in the sense of the loss of orientation. I don't know at all where I am in the world. Gur Aryeh says that this is a universal. It's a very common reaction to a situation in which one is almost—almost—almost... [T]he reaction is a sense of theological vertigo, of asking what does anything mean in that case. If it's really just a matter of a millimeter—it could go this way, it could go that way—how do we understand God's providence? How do we understand anything, in view of such events? The interesting thing is that Rashi, as interpreted by the Maharal (and Rashi is *the* classic interpreter of the Bible), indicates that Sarah dies of something like this. She does not die thinking that Isaac is dead. She knows he's alive, but only by a hair's breadth. And that immediately sets everything awry, does something radical to her sense of order and coherence in

the world.[1]

Sarah, on this read, could not live in a world so stripped of meaning and reliability. Her son's life was no longer a given. God's protection was no longer a given. Fairness was no longer a given. Maybe her husband's sanity or compassion or character were no longer givens. Her sense of stability was undone completely. And the result was profound disorientation. Life could not go on. Everything was off kilter once presented with the harsh reality of a seemingly arbitrary universe. Sarah's physical death, then, reflected or performed the death of her world as she knew it.

Zornberg's poetic term "theological vertigo" captures this deeply existential notion that loss—or *almost*-loss—destabilizes and calls into question our sense of order or coherence in the world. It rattles our very beings, shakes us from complaisance, mocks our sense of safety. It is said that disease causes dis-ease. As Sarah shows us, it can also cause death: not only death of bodies, but also the collapse of internal worlds.

It seems to me that the pandemic of Covid-19 has pushed all of us to live in close proximity to death, to viscerally and continually contend with the hair's breadth that stands between wellness and illness, order and disorder, coherence and incoherence. It is but a *davar muat*—one very small, microscopic thing—that keeps us vital and our world functional. We live in liminal space, really knowing the precarity of it all. And that is a very dizzying consciousness. Theological vertigo just might be the all-too-human condition that accompanies the viral disease.

Is there a medicine for this malaise? How might we live in the face of such rupture and disorientation? Sarah's personal story does not augur well. Some will tragically be lost to the experience of almost-loss. But Jewish history is anchored in collective loss and it is characterized by collective resilience, so there are resources that we might draw upon to find our grounding once again.

The destruction of the second Temple in Jerusalem in 70 CE, for example, was a rupture of the highest order. The house of God was destroyed; the nexus of communal gathering laid waste; the majestic emblem of a

---

[1] Avivah Gottlieb Zornberg, "Cries and Whispers: The Death of Sarah," in *Beginning Anew: A Woman's Companion to the High Holy Days*, edited by Gail Twersky Reimer and Judith A. Kates, (New York: Touchstone, 1997), 182-183.

culture wrecked. It was a loss that is still grieved to this day. So devastated were those who lived through it, that it was not clear that life itself could continue, or ought to, amidst such absence.

Babylonian Talmud, Baba Batra 60b, relays one conversation to this effect:

> Our Rabbis taught: When the Temple was destroyed for the second time, large numbers [of people in] Israel became ascetics, binding themselves neither to eat meat nor to drink wine. R. Joshua got into a conversation with them and said to them: My sons, why do you not eat meat nor drink wine? They replied: Shall we eat flesh which used to be brought as an offering on the altar, now that this altar is in abeyance? Shall we drink wine which used to be poured as a libation on the altar, but now no longer? He said to them: If that is so, we should not eat bread either, because the meal offerings have ceased. They said: [That is so, and] we can manage with fruit. We should not eat fruit either, [he said,] because there is no longer an offering of first fruits. Then we can manage with other fruits [they said]. But, [he said,] we should not drink water, because there is no longer any ceremony of the pouring of water. To this they could find no answer.

> So he said to them: My sons, come and listen to me. Not to mourn at all is impossible, because the blow has fallen. To mourn overmuch is also impossible, because we do not impose on the community a hardship which the majority cannot endure.

> The Sages therefore have ordained thus. A man may stucco his house, but he should leave a little [davar muat] bare... A man can prepare a full-course banquet, but he should leave out an item or two [davar muat]... A woman can put on all her ornaments, but leave off one or two [davar muat]. For so it says, If I forget thee, O Jerusalem, let my right hand forget, let my tongue cleave to the roof of my mouth if I remember

thee not, if I prefer not Jerusalem above my chief joy. What is meant by "my chief joy"? R. Isaac said: This is symbolized by the burnt ashes which we place on the head of a bridegroom.

In the face of destabilizing loss, there are those who may wish to retreat or give up—to step away from food, away from nourishment, away from life, as the ascetics in this story suggest. But the Sages offer an alternative: to step back into life—to build, to feast, to celebrate, to seduce—and to do so in ways that *contain* loss, while also *retaining* it. Four laws are introduced to this effect. When constructing a house, one ought to leave one small area unplastered or unpainted. When hosting a banquet, one ought to leave one dish off the menu. When dressing up, one ought to leave off one ornament. Finally, when getting married, ashes ought to be placed on the forehead of the groom. In these ways, one might consciously keep alive the awareness of incompletion in one's home, table, body, or relationships without being hollowed out by it. One can keep brokenness—and all of its hard-won truths—at the forefront of one's consciousness without being broken by it.

The Talmudic language of *davar muat,* a small thing, is noteworthy, as it brings us back to the Maharal on Sarah. He writes, "*Davar muat haya shelo nishchat,*" it was just a small thing that kept Isaac from being slaughtered and just a small thing that caused Sarah's demise. Here that same awareness is on display—awareness of the hair's breadth that separates life and death, coherence and incoherence, vitality and torpidity. But the rabbis charge nevertheless to continue to live, to paint, to eat, to dress up, to love. Just leave off a little bit.

When our worlds fall apart, our instincts might be to withdraw, but this tradition asks us to find a way to accommodate a new reality—one that actively but subtly incorporates the consciousness of *davar muat;* one that affirms the truth of instability, yet is not incapacitated by it. This might be one way to find solid ground in the throes of vertigo.

* * *

What follows is a collection of reflections on these vertiginous times and various attempts at finding balance. Some of us don't build homes, after all, to find stability. (Some of us don't even leave our homes.) Some of us seek stability through words, through history, through solidarity, through a Jewish tradition that reminds us time and again that our "unprecedented" times have much precedent. From the ten plagues of the Bible through the Bubonic Plague of the Middle Ages, Talmudic *magefah* misfortunes to shtetl outbreaks and beyond, the Jewish people—alongside the rest of humanity—has suffered through a great deal of disruptive adversity. *Torah in a Time of Plague* brings together academic and rabbinic voices from within the Covid-19 plague to wrestle in real time with its echoes and implications.

Section 1, *Theology of Plague,* reckons with some of the many theological disturbances that the pandemic has wrought: challenges of randomness (Magid, Tucker); of making sense of a loving God in a broken world (Sabath Beit-Halachmi, Richman, Schoenfeld, Green); human responsibility versus divine culpability in the face of disaster (Kalman and Seidler-Feller). Here are contemporary reckonings with the age-old problem of theodicy.

Section 2, *Jewish Community and Practice Under Duress,* takes up issues related to ritual, law, and collective activity that have arisen on account of the social dictates of Covid-19. Quarantines and full lockdowns characterized the early months of the pandemic and continue to determine if we gather, how we gather (Labaton), where we gather (Aranoff), and what religious acts we might perform individually or together (Libson, Jacobson-Maisels). They have certainly prodded us to re-evaluate the meaning and power of gathering (Mayse, Levisohn). These essays offer insights into the stresses of aloneness and the yearning for togetherness that has marked this time.

Section 3, *History and Literature of Plague,* turns to plagues of the past to see how they affected their European Jewish communities. Using liturgy (Landes) and responsa literature (Teplitsky), we can see how grave illness yielded tremendous physical loss, altered religious life, and also generated creativity.

Section 4, *Quarantine Reflections,* invites some personal meditations on the costs and gifts of Covid-19. From giving birth amidst relentless death (Tweel) to raising and reading with children (Kurshan); celebrating the Sabbath in isolation to studying Tractate Shabbat with a virtual global community (Leib), these essays attest to the complexities of our everyday lives in lockdown.

Finally, Section 5, *Time in Unprecedented Times,* explores the ways that time itself has been warped by the plague of our age. Thrust into our homes and out of our routines, Covid-19 has altered how we relate to temporality (Atkins). Time bends, shrinks, and expands when the schedules that anchored our lives are no longer our signposts. The passage of time in our bodies, aging, has also taken on new meanings as we reckon with feelings of "lost time" (Fishbane).

Torah in a Time of Plague both reflects on and contributes to Torah in our time. As we continue to navigate our way through the multi-layered coronavirus epidemic, let these eclectic, sobering, and stirring writings be "small things" that help us find a way through the vertigo.

Erin Leib Smokler
January 2021

The Theology of Plague

Covid-19 and the Theological
Challenge of the Arbitrary

Shaul Magid

"Science doesn't think"
—Martin Heidegger

Religion's use and interpretation of natural phenomena and catastrophes as indications of divine favor or wrath has a long history.[1] We need look no further than the first ten chapters of Genesis to see two natural phenomena, the flood and the rainbow, as illustrations.

Looking more deeply into the Hebrew Bible, we are confronted with two other natural phenomena, famine and plagues, as turning points in Israelite history.[2] A famine caused Abraham and then Jacob to travel to Egypt, and plagues mark a transition whereby God intervenes directly to liberate the Israelites from slavery.[3] A famine initiated what would become Israelite exile, and a series of plagues initiated the Israelites' redemption from Egypt. In the Hebrew Bible, and in the ancient world more gener-

---

[1] See, for example, D. K. Chester, "The Theodicy of Natural Disasters," Scottish Journal of Theology 51, no. 4 (1998): 485–505. Cf. Charles Rosenberg, The Cholera Years: The United States in 1832, 1849, and 1866 (Chicago, 1987), 4–64; and Lori Veilleux, "Religion and Disaster: A Case of Boston's Response to the 1832 Cholera Epidemic" (PhD diss., Brown University, 2014); and J. C. Gaillard, "Religions, Natural Hazards, and Disasters: An Introduction," Religion 40, no. 2 (2101): 81–84.

[2] There are numerous terms used in the Hebrew Bible to refer to plagues, for example, magafah, dever, and to a lesser extent makah. Makah is most often used to refer to human generated acts of violence, but also sometimes refers to plague-like acts of God, such as in 1 Samuel 6:19, ". . . for the same plague (makah) struck all of you and your lords." In terms of magafah, see 1 Samuel 4:17, where the JPS Tanakh translates it as "slaughter," but 1 Samuel 6:4, where it is translated as "plague." Psalms 106:29 says, "They provoked anger by their deeds, and a plague (magafah) broke out among them." In most of the cases where magafah and makah are used, they refer to divine decrees in response to bad behavior. The term dever, which is used to describe the plagues in Egypt, is the one used in the Babylonian Talmud. This term seems to imply something that is not directly the result of recalcitrance.

[3] In the story of the Egyptian plagues, both dever and magafah are used. For example, Exodus 9:3, 14. In 9:3, magafah is translated as "plague" and in 9:14 dever is translated as "pestilence."

ally, plagues and famine are major occurrences that initiate demographic shifts. In the Bible and other religious texts, there is often a direct correlation between God and natural phenomena. The ancients' view of famine was quite comprehensible, as there was an empirical connection between drought and famine. They knew *how* famines occurred, even if they did not know why, although the assumption was that they were punishments for human sin.

Famines constitute a good portion of the mishnaic tractate Ta'anit, and are viewed in the mishnah largely as a divine punishment. Thus, the mishnah mandates fasting and repentance to nullify the decree. The famous story of the first-century *tanna* (teacher), Honi Ha-me'agel, drawing a circle in which he sat and prayed for rain personifies the notion that famine was viewed as a consequence of human wrongdoing and thus required human correction.[4]

Plagues were much more ambiguous. The plagues in Egypt had a clear and explicit teleological function: to break the will of the Egyptians in order to convince Pharaoh to free the Jews. These plagues are described in the exegetical tradition as targeted—only affecting the Egyptians—with the plague of the firstborn being the culminating, and explicit, example. In short, these phenomena fit neatly into a world where God intervenes in nature to achieve certain ends.[5]

Plagues as described in the Babylonian Talmud, however, seem to suggest something different. There is one talmudic *sugya* (passage from the Gemarah) devoted to plagues (*dever*), b. Bava Kama 60b, that is almost entirely concerned with ways to best protect oneself from contagion.[6] There is no mention there of praying, repenting, fasting, or engaging in other devotional acts to ward off the disease. Medieval commentators on this *sugya* mostly reflect on the arbitrariness of a plague, which does not seem to be something that can be undone by devotional acts and contrition.[7]

---

[4] b. Ta'anit 23a.

[5] On the distinction between the plagues in Egypt and a general plague, see Rabbi Shmuel Eidels (the Maharsha), *Hiddushei Aggadot*, on Bava Kama 60b in standard editions of the Babylonian Talmud. His commentary is included in the back of standard editions of the Talmud and is not published separately.

[6] There are only two references to magafot in the Babylonian Talmud: Moed Katan 28a and Sotah 44b (both are passing references). The term dever is used for the Babylonian Talmud's sustained discussion on plagues.

[7] See, for example, in *Sefer Or Zaruah* 2.407 discussing b. Ta'anit 19b in regard to whether

Below, I argue that the Babylonian Talmud's one extended discussion of *dever* in b. Bava Kama 60b resists the notion of collapsing plagues into covenantal categories, whereby we can see them as acts of divine intervention to punish evildoers, Jews or non-Jews. Rather, as we will see in several glosses to the talmudic *sugya*, plagues seem to be arbitrary occurrences, indiscriminate, and thus impervious to human devotional intervention. In this sense, they are extra-covenantal occurrences challenging rabbinic convention that natural disasters are in some way divine intervention to punish or facilitate a response.

Plagues present an interesting case of what I am calling a "covenantal exception" that is both problematic and necessary. While the arbitrary poses certain theological challenges to covenantal reciprocity (if plagues are arbitrary, what are the limits of the arbitrary?), the arbitrary also serves a crucial function as exception. Without the notion of the arbitrary as extra-covenantal, Judaism becomes vulnerable to making all disasters, even those that equally affect non-Jews, the fault of the Jews, which could easily, and understandably, evoke negative reactions. Plague as the exception thus enables Jews to understand natural disasters outside the paradigm of reward and punishment.

There is a distinction I want to draw here between arbitrariness and uncertainty (*safek*), the latter being a major category of halakhic discourse.[8] In his recent book *The Birth of Doubt*, Moshe Halbertal gives us two operative models of uncertainty in rabbinic literature. First, the uncertainty concerning reality. This sometimes has multiple levels. One example Halbertal brings is from Mishnah Shabbat: when a wall falls on Shabbat and one doesn't know if there are people under the rubble; or, if there are, whether they are alive or dead. This raises halakhic questions as to whether one is permitted, or even obligated, to transgress Sabbath law to dig through the rubble under the aegis of *pikuah nefesh* (saving a life). The second category is uncertainty about a rule, that is, which rule should apply in any given circumstance. Halbertal argues that *safek* is thus not a marginal halakhic circumstance, but it is woven into the halakhic

---

one can or should fast or pray during a plague.

[8] Moshe Halbertal, *The Birth of Doubt: Confronting Uncertainty in Early Rabbinic Literature* (Providence, RI: Brown Judaica Series, 2020).

system itself.[9]

Arbitrariness finds no real roots in halakhah because it challenges the entire covenantal system. Halakhah requires either a realm of certainty (that is, this is the reality, so what shall be done?) or of doubt *about* that reality, such that uncertainty can be adjudicated to satisfy conformity to rabbinic norms. In either case, the theological question of *why* the wall fell on Shabbat is not addressed in the mishnah. Halbertal's two models do not present any overt theological challenges but rather practical ones concerning how to properly behave when uncertainty inserts itself into a situation.

Arbitrariness, however, is arguably all about a theological challenge. In some way, arbitrariness is the epitome of heresy, as the rabbis articulate heresy through the adage "there is no judge and there is no judgment (*leit din ve-leit dayan*)."[10] One way of understanding this is to say, "everything is arbitrary." This, of course, is quite different than saying "*some* things are arbitrary," which gives rise to the notion of "the world acts according to its manner" (*olam kemin-hago noheg*), a rabbinic dictum that is used in a very limited way in talmudic literature, but one which Moses Maimonides expands to define nature more generally.[11] Yet, I suggest the notion of a self-generating nature is not the same as arbitrariness in regard to plagues, which do not seem to be part of a normal, and thus somewhat predictable, cycle. It is precisely the extra-ordinary, be it miracles or, in our case, plagues, when divine agency seems to be at work.[12] And yet, as we will see, the plagues described in b. Bava Kama 60b appear to exist outside any frame of a covenantal system.

I proceed below by offering a series of medieval examples by talmudic glossators who reflect on the unspoken notion that *dever* are not phenomena that require fasting and prayer to nullify the decree because they

---

[9] See Halbertal, *The Birth of Doubt*, 2–3.

[10] On the heresy of Elisha ben Avuyah and the notion of erasing the covenant, see Alon Goshen-Gottstein, *The Sinner and the Amnesiac: The Rabbinic Invention of Elisha ben Avuyah and Elazar ben Arach* (Stanford: Stanford University Press, 2000). See also Yehuda Liebes, Heto shel Elisha (Jerusalem: Magnus Press, 1990).

[11] See, for example, in b. Avodah Zarah 54b. Maimonides uses the term in many places, in an expansive mode in relation to nature; see his Eight Chapters, chapter 8.

[12] Maimonides uses the saying "the world acts according to its manner" as a way of explaining miracles in *The Guide to the Perplexed* 2.29. It is, however, the only time that saying is used in the Guide.

appear to exist outside the covenant framework.

The talmudic *sugya* in b. Bava Kama 60b reads as follows:

> The Sages taught: If there is plague in the city, gather your feet,
> that is, limit the time you spend out of the house, as it is stated
> in the verse: "And none of you shall go out of the opening of
> his house until the morning" (Exodus 12:22). And it says in
> another verse: "Come, my people, enter into your chambers,
> and shut your doors behind you; hide yourself for a little
> moment, until the anger has passed by" (Isaiah 26:20). And
> it says: "Outside the sword will bereave, and in the chambers
> terror" (Deuteronomy 32:25) . . . At a time when there was
> a plague, Rava would close the windows of his house, as it is
> written: "For death is come up into our windows" (Jeremiah
> 9:20). The Sages taught: If there is famine in the city, spread
> your feet, that is, leave the city, as it is stated in the verse: "And
> there was a famine in the land; and Abram went down into
> Egypt to sojourn there" (Genesis 12:10). And it says: "If we say:
> We will enter into the city, then the famine is in the city, and we
> shall die there; and if we sit here, we die also, now come, and
> let us fall unto the host of the Arameans; if they save us alive,
> we shall live; and if they kill us, we shall but die" (2 Kings 7:4)
> . . . The Sages taught: If there is a plague in the city, a person
> should not walk in the middle of the road, due to the fact that
> the angel of death walks in the middle of the road, as, since in
> heaven they have given him permission to kill within the city,
> he goes openly in the middle of the road. By contrast, if there
> is peace and quiet in the city, do not walk on the sides of the
> road, as, since the angel of death does not have permission to
> kill within the city, he hides himself and walks on the side of
> the road.[13]

In Rabbi Bezalel Ashkenazi's (1520–92) *Shitah Me-kubetset* (Gathered
Interpretation) to Bava Kama 60b we read the following:

---

[13] Unless otherwise noted, all translations are mine.

When there is a plague in the city, a person should not enter the synagogue alone because the angel of death places his vessels there, as it says, "At Michmash he deposited his baggage" (Isaiah 10:25). This is difficult to understand. How does this verse prove anything? It seems to me that he only brings them to the synagogue because this verse is dealing with Sanharev (Sennacherib), who passed by all the places mentioned in Isaiah and, when he reached the city of Michmash, he left his vessels there because he didn't need to bring all his weapons into battle since he knew he would win anyway. So, too, the angel of death at a time of a plague; he doesn't need all his weapons because he was already given permission to destroy, so he leaves them there and goes on.[14]

The notion that "the angel of death at a time of a plague doesn't need all his weapons because he was already given permission to destroy" suggests that a plague represents a time of arbitrary destruction through the unleashed power of the angel of death, not as a means of punishment for Israel's sins. Empirically, of course, this is evident; plagues do not pinpoint certain groups and exclude others (contra the tradition's understanding of the plagues in Egypt) and, as opposed to natural disasters, they are not viewed as inevitable consequences of nature, nor are they geographically limited. Thus, the notion of the targeted plagues in Egypt—clearly targeted as acts of punishment—are really counter examples to the way the Babylonian Talmud seems to understand plagues in general.

The Babylonian Talmud's focus is on avoiding contagion rather trying to nullify it. In Rabbi Shlomo Luria's (1510–73) *Yam Shel Shlomo* (Sea of Solomon) we read a reflection on the talmudic advice to flee a city where there is a plague:

We also say, all roads have the status of a dangerous place (*kheskat sakanah*). Thus, it is not advised to flee [the city], especially after the plague strengthens. There is a greater danger to one who flees in regard to the other nations [who may rob him], than to flee the plague, as is known, according

---

[14] *Shitah Me-kubetset* to Bava Kama, 107b–c.

to our sins. However, at the outset [of the plague] it is good to flee . . . we know that Rava did not flee. Maybe it was because he knew it wouldn't help.[15]

Noteworthy here is the seeming arbitrary nature of a plague, which makes those who seek to flee vulnerable to human criminality. Perhaps Rava stayed where he was because he knew fleeing "wouldn't help," that is, he took his chances with contagion as opposed to endangering himself by becoming vulnerable to thievery. As was the case in b. Bava Kama 60b, there is no mention in Luria of prayer, repentance, or fasting to avert the danger. Therefore, like the talmudic *sugya* itself, it appears these commentators also view a plague as an arbitrary occurrence. Most glossators on the *sugya* in the Babylonian Talmud follow the Talmud's logic that a plague is something that requires diligent avoidance and not any attempt to nullify the decree through pious behavior. This is in stark contrast to famine, where the mishnaic sages and their interpreters engage in programmatic procedures to nullify the decree through acts of penance. A similar approach can be found in Nahmanides' gloss to Ta'anit 22b and Rabbi Menachem Ha-Meiri's (1249-1310) gloss to Ta'anit 22b where there is a distinction made between a *dever* and a famine or collapsed building (*mefolet*).

My claim here is that the oddity and theological danger of plagues being arbitrary acts of unbridled evil does not pass by later sages unnoticed, and yet each maintains plagues as distinct from famine or collapsed buildings in regard to fasting and penance. There seems to be a gentle but persistent resistance to what is implied in the *sugya*, while the basic distinction of arbitrariness is never openly challenged. I say implied because the Talmud does not openly make the claim of arbitrariness, but in its suggestions for escaping the plague it never yields to penance the way it does with famines. That is, it does not offer what would be a predictable response that would include both physical avoidance and acts geared toward nullification.

Below, I provide three examples that seem to counter—or at least resist—both the rabbinic text and earlier glossators in viewing the *sugya*'s discussion of *dever* as aligned with a more classic notion of misfortune

---

[15] Shlomo Luria, Yam Shel Shlomo, DBS Master Library: The Most Complete Judaic Library, Version 12.0 - 662 Sifrei Kodesh [CD-ROM].

as a product of human fallibility. My suggestion is that these illustrate an anxiety produced by the description of an event that stands outside the covenantal paradigm of reward and punishment, in part because it raises the question of how one can ascertain what is and is not an arbitrary occurrence.

In Rabbi Moshe Cordovero's (1522–70) *Pardes Rimonim* (Orchard of Pomegranates) 8:1, we read the following:

> The Zohar says that at the time of a plague, heaven forbid, a person should cover their forehead so that the angel of death will not recognize his sins that are engraved on his forehead. Hence, the rabbis teach us, everyone who drinks wine and eats meat on Erev Tisha b'Av, his sins will be engraved on his bones, as it says, "And their sins will be upon your bones" (Ezekiel 32:27).[16]

Cordovero, citing the Zohar, views a plague as comparable to any other natural disaster: as punishment for sin. He thus advises his reader to act appropriately while also suggesting that, if the angel of death does not *see* sin, the angel will "pass over" the individual, in a sense squaring plagues in general with the plagues in Egypt—specifically the plague of the first born, where Israel was asked to mark their doorposts so that the angel of death would pass them by. Of course, here it is the opposite. Cordovero asks his reader to conceal his identity as a sinner so that the plague will not visit his/her home. With this he implies that a contemporary plague is no different than its biblical antecedents. The interesting thing is that the *sugya* could have easily made such a prescription yet chose not to.

A second example comes from Rabbi Yitzhak Arama's (1420–94) *Akedat Yitshak* (Binding of Isaac), gate 26, where we see a similar yet more muted approach:

> When there is a plague in the city, "gather your feet." Why should one be outside when the angel of death stands in the streets of the city? If we see that things are getting worse, flee quickly to a quiet and safe place. If it finds him even in

---

[16] Cordovero, *Pardes Rimonim* (Jerusalem, 1962), 35 a–b.

that place, he should take any and all medications that can prolong his life. In most cases that will suffice. And if this is not successful, he will have fulfilled his obligation to do everything to save himself and he will know that it is God who sent this angel [of death] and there is no escape from it. What else can he do but prepare for his death and draw from all his merit? He should use this to try to turn to God. This should be done in all such similar cases that come to the world.[17]

Once again, there is no mention of prayer, repentance, or fasting, but only taking all medical precautions. And yet, the covenantal frame gently returns when Arama says, "he will know that it is God who sent this angel [of death] and there is no escape from it." Although Arama recommends that the reader turn to God, this turning seems more a preparation for death than an effort to avert the plague. Arama does link the angel of death to God, something that is not done, for example, in Bezalel Ashkenazi's gloss. Arama's comment here is a good example of one who responds to rabbinic silence on the plague as punishment by interjecting a covenantal frame as a way to square the talmudic dicta with more conventional thinking.

Finally, Rabbi Moshe Alshekh's (1508–93) *Commentary to Ecclesiastes* 8:7 offers us yet another example. Alshekh begins with the assumption that human beings (he doesn't distinguish between Jew and non-Jew) are protected, or sometimes made vulnerable, by astrological constellations. Therefore, even if one's astrological fate is that he or she be killed in a plague, why should another, whose fate is dictated by another constellation, also fall victim to this fate? It's not clear if he is asking why one's constellation does not protect them from another's. Alshekh makes the following assertion:

Why is it that when there is a plague, so many people die? Isn't it possible for one to avoid being a victim to this by being overseen by [being ruled over by] another constellation? Maybe you will say the constellation of the many overrides the constellation of the few, which will result in the death of

17 Yitzhak Arama, *Akedat Yitshak*, gate 26, DBS Master Library.

one's brethren? There is another example we can give from war. If the constellation that oversees a king destines that he should fall, why should his soldiers and thousands of others, whose time has not come, also fall? And why should the protection of [that is, granted by] other constellations be nullified for another? Rather, it is certainly the case that this is all from heaven.[18]

Reaching back to the ancient notion of constellations dictating earthly phenomena and human destiny, Alshekh asks directly about the arbitrariness of plagues.[19] If one person, or a group, merits death by a plague, what about those outside the sphere of punishment? It is the classic question of what we might call "collateral damage." Refraining from responding to the perennial question of arbitrary death, Alshekh ends simply with, "it is certainly the case that this is all from heaven." Without coming up with an answer to his own questions, Alshekh resorts to a pious retort of everything being determined by God, thus suggesting that while plagues do seem to be mysterious in their arbitrariness they must be, in the end, divinely ordained, even if they seem indiscriminate. While I am not sure when Alshekh wrote his commentary, he and Cordovero lived in Safed during a series of devastating plagues, one of which, in 1572, killed kabbalist Isaac Luria at the young age of 38, ending a career that began only two years earlier but was already revolutionizing Kabbalah.[20] That plague severely damaged the Jewish community, causing many to emigrate to other locales.

In any case, I suggest that what we witness here in these final three

---

[18] Moshe Alshekh, *Commentary to Ecclesiastes* 8:7, DBS Master Library.

[19] Ancient Jewish astrology is a giant field of research, and the belief that individuals and communities were tied to astrological constellations was common in ancient Judaism. For two examples, see Annette Yoshiko Reed, "'Ancient Jewish Sciences' and the Historiography of Judaism," in *Ancient Jewish Sciences and the History of Knowledge in Second Temple Literature*, ed. Jonathan Ben-Dov and Seth Sanders (New York: NYU Press, 2014), 195–254, and Jeffrey L. Rubenstein, "Talmudic Astrology, Bavli Šabbat 156a–b," *Hebrew Union College Annual* 78 (2007): 109–48.

[20] On Safed in the sixteenth century and plagues, see Abraham David, *To Come to the Land: Immigration and Settlement in 16th Century Eretz-Israel*, trans. Dena Ordan. (Tuscaloosa, AL: University of Alabama Press, 1999), and David Tamar, *Aliyah ve-hityashvut be-erets Yisrael be-meah ha-shishit* (Jerusalem: Reuven Mass, 1993).

examples—Cordovero, Arama, and Alshekh—is the tension with, and resistance to, the talmudic sages and some of its commentators who suggest that plagues are non-covenantal phenomena: for example, by treating the plague as the free rein of the angel of death, regardless of one's behavior. This appears to be the way Bezalel Ashkenazi and Shlomo Luria interpret the talmudic passage. Such arbitrariness seems dissonant to Cordovero, Arama, and Alshekh, who each try to fit this phenomenon of the arbitrary into a more normative covenantal frame. Perhaps these attempts simply beg the question of whether the indiscriminate nature of plagues—expressed succinctly in Bezalel Ashkenazi's comment about the ways they unleash the free rein of the angel of death—is something that tests the very limits of a covenantal paradigm.

Part of this may be a response to the mysteriousness of plagues. Famine is tangible and understandable, but if we look at how ancient and medieval Jewish sources relate to plagues, specifically Bava Kama 60b which is the Talmud's most sustained discussion, it appears the authors of this *sugya* and their glossators knew that people were getting sick, but they didn't really know how or why. They certainly knew empirically that plagues and their contagion were indiscriminate; Jews, non-Jews, righteous and wicked, all fell ill. Thus, with regard to the age-old theodicy question that goes back to Job—"Why do the wicked prosper and the righteous suffer?"—a plague's indiscriminate nature doesn't quite allow that frame to become operative, since righteous and wicked seem to be affected equally.

Whereas the question of God's role in human catastrophes like the Holocaust abound, the sages do not ask similar questions in relation to plagues. The Holocaust is a question of human evil, and thus, the theological questions revolve around God's participation in, or absence from, that evil. Asking the question of theodicy is, therefore, precarious on two fronts. First, it potentially implicates God in acts of evil; and second, it potentially absents God from acts of evil, thereby limiting, or threatening, the covenantal paradigm.

The theological challenge of something like Covid-19 is precisely the challenge the Sages saw in plagues. The inadvertent and indiscriminate nature of plagues pushes the covenantal paradigm to its very limits. I think this tension appears in the way some of the later authorities we examined try to "covenantize" the arbitrary. That is, they try to square indiscriminate death with some notion of reward and punishment that in some way, even though a plague appears to function outside any covenantal frame, makes the plague no different than the way the Sages understood famine in Tractate Ta'anit: as a divine intervention caused by Israel's sin. What is curious is that the Talmud does not seem to treat plagues that way, at least not in Bava Kama 60b.

Something like the Holocaust is more understandable, albeit even less fathomable. This is because we can, sadly, understand the depravity of human evil ("for the intent of man's heart is evil from his youth," Genesis 8:21) even if we can't quite fathom how God permitted such evil to do such damage. The theological question of the Holocaust revolves around how God could have enabled human beings to be *that* successful in murdering Jews.[21] With plagues, there is no subject to which we can point other than an invisible microbe whose only purpose is its own survival. The Sages, interestingly, do not point to God as the source but focus instead on the pragmatics of avoiding contagion. Later sources try to fit the arbitrary into a more compelling, and in some sense, more comfortable covenantal box—that is, they evoke God to mute the arbitrary. Examples include comments like the plague "must be from heaven" or asking Jews to cover their forehead so the angel of death will not see the sins that are emblazoned there.

I suggested here that the tension of the arbitrary as it threatens the covenantal paradigm is exhibited by the later attempts to fit it into the relationship between God and Israel. Yet, this attempt to curb the arbitrary comes with a cost. The danger of Jews taking a clearly indiscriminate occurrence like a plague and viewing it in some ways as part of a reciprocal relationship between God and Israel carries with it a serious downside. We know, for example, that Jews were often blamed for natural disasters, including plagues. The antisemitism of the medieval church often used natural disasters as a way to stoke their theological anti-Jewish beliefs, and considerable anti-Jewish violence often accompanied such tragedies.[22]

---

[21] This informs the work of Richard Rubenstein in *After Auschwitz* (first published in 1966), and informs almost all post-Holocaust theology in its wake. The post-Holocaust theological question is about human evil and divine agency. What is at stake is not that human beings could implement genocide, but how God could allow it.

[22] See Susan Einbinder, *After the Black Death: Plague and Commemoration Among Iberian Jews* (Philadelphia: University of Pennsylvania Press, 2019), 14–31.

We know the histories of how Jews were implicated in the Black Death in the fourteenth century. Many clerical figures also blamed this plague on the sins of their Christian constituents. In Spain, the Jews as "killers of Christ" became predictable victims. In Germany and France, rumors soon spread that Jews were engaged in poisoning wells—that is, it was not just that they were sinners for rejecting Christ, but that they were actively behind the spread of the plague.[23]

While, historically, Jews were blamed for things about which they were clearly not responsible, theologically, the covenantal frame that supports Judaism's sense of both its destiny as well as its notion of divine election clearly carries with it some occupational hazards. It is one thing for Jews to blame themselves for atrocities that happen to them—for example, the destruction of the Jerusalem temples. It is quite another thing for Jews to blame themselves for disasters that happen to them as well as others around them, such as natural disasters. Trying to fit what is ostensibly arbitrary into a covenantal framework, whereby Jews are the cause of such a disaster, can potentially evoke anti-Jewish feelings among others who also suffer from those disasters. While there may be an inclination among Jews to view such events as a response to their sins, there is an equally powerful inclination to refrain from doing so. Such covenantal responses could easily be used to blame the Jews, who have historically been suspect in many of the societies in which they lived.[24]

In this reading, the arbitrary is both theologically problematic and yet a crucial component of the Jews' understanding of the world and their place in it. By acknowledging the arbitrary, Jews concede that not everything that happens to them is the result of their covenantal relationship with God. By acknowledging this, they must then navigate how and when the arbitrary works, and what its criteria and limits are. To overextend the arbitrary can easily yield to the classic rabbinic doctrine of heresy, "there is no judge and there is not judgment," cited above. In a sense, this kind of Jewish heresy is the maximization of the arbitrary. On the other hand,

---

[23] For a synopsis, see Dan Freedman, "Why Were Jews Blamed for the Black Death?" *Moment Magazine*, Mar. 31, 2000, https://momentmag.com/why-were-jews-blamed-for-the-black-death/. Cf. Samuel K. Cohn, "The Black Death and the Burning of the Jews," Past and Present 196, no. 1 (Aug. 2007): 3–36.

[24] See, for example, David Nirenberg, *Anti-Judaism: The Western Tradition* (New York: W.W. Norton and Company, 2013), esp. 87–134 and 183–17.

by viewing everything that happens to Jews—especially when those very same things happen to others—as the fault of Jews, Jews open themselves to being blamed for the calamities that other people experience. And thus, as Jonah said to his compatriots on the ship in stormy seas, if you just throw me overboard, you will be saved.[25] They did so, and they were saved.

It seems to me that all this was not lost in the sources we cited in regard to plagues. On the one hand, we need to keep the arbitrary intact so that Jews will be considered as much innocent victims of plagues as any other group. And, on the other hand, later sources feel understandably uncomfortable with the arbitrary and what it might mean in terms of covenantal theology more generally.

One can see a more contemporary example in the way post-Holocaust theologians like Eliezer Berkovitz resisted Richard Rubenstein's removal of God from the Holocaust.[26] If God was *not* a party to the Holocaust, how can the covenant survive? And if God *was* a party to the Holocaust, what kind of God can survive? In fact, one could argue that the battle lines in post-Holocaust theology are largely drawn around the question of whether the covenant—and God—can sustain the absence of God in the Holocaust.[27] The Holocaust as an act of human depravity, of course, was not arbitrary at all but rather a highly calculated act. The point of comparison is only that in both cases, whether a plague or the Holocaust, God is absent and, thus, the act or event cannot be viewed as a case of divine intervention.

Covid-19, like all plagues, will subside as a pandemic. But what we have experienced these last months is nothing less than a global plague that may be distinctive because with worldwide travel, a contagion can reach around the planet in a very short time. The social, political, and humanitarian challenges loom large and the human devastation is significant. What is given less attention are the theological challenges such natural catastrophes present to communities of faith. This too deserves our attention. When the plague passes and we move back to a relatively

---

[25] Jonah 1:12.

[26] See, for example, Eliezer Berkovitz, *Faith After the Holocaust* (Jerusalem: Maggid Press, 2019).

[27] See, for example, Zachary Braiterman, *(God) After Auschwitz* (Princeton: Princeton University Press, 1998), 19–34, and Barbara Krawcowicz, *History, Metahistory, and Evil: Jewish Theological Responses to the Holocaust* (Boston: Academic Studies Press, 2020).

normal way of life, the more concrete challenges of human survival will dissipate. But the theological challenges the arbitrary introduces, and the extent to which we are willing to engage them, will remain.

Theodicy and the Slings and Arrows
of Outrageous Fortune

Gordon Tucker

We are living now in a time of a calamitous pandemic plague. Historically, when such catastrophic events have inflicted themselves on human lives and societies, theology has often shifted into a mode known as theodicy. Its aim is generally twofold: to uphold the idea of divine control of events, and, crucially, to justify that divine involvement in the disasters.[1] In other words, two conceptual aversions combine to drive theodicy: (1) to contingency and randomness,[2] and (2) to an ascription of amorality (not to mention *immorality*) to actions or inactions of the deity.[3]

Here is how Kant defined theodicy:

> By "theodicy" we understand the defense of the highest wisdom of the creator against the charge which reason brings against it for whatever is counterpurposive in the world.[4]

Given all of this, it is natural to assume that this defense of the Creator is a quintessentially pious endeavor. Proposed theodicies have, in fact, suffered a rocky history, with respect to their perceived validity and per-

---

[1] A single example will suffice to illustrate what is a ubiquitous biblical phenomenon: "Why is the land in ruins, laid waste like a wilderness, with none passing through? The Lord replied: Because they forsook the Teaching I had set before them"—Jer. 9:11-12.

[2] Although these terms (contingency and randomness) do not always denote the same thing, I will be using them more or less interchangeably. They are meant to express the notion that there are manifold phenomena and events in the world that do not follow inexorably from prior states of the world (or from the divine will), and could readily have been otherwise than they are.

[3] As H.L. Ginsberg pointed out in his introduction to the Book of Lamentations in *The Five Megilloth and Jonah* (Jewish Publication Society of America 1969, p. 33), even though the author does not know the nature of the transgression(s), "Our poems...express certainty that Jerusalem must have sinned grievously," i.e., there is nothing random or amoral about the devastation lamented in the book.

[4] Immanuel Kant, "On the Miscarriage of All Philosophical Trials in Theodicy," in *Religion Within the Boundaries of Mere Reason and Other Writings*, trans. Allen Wood (Cambridge: Cambridge University Press, 2018), 31.

suasiveness. But the piety of the intentions behind theodicy has generally not been doubted.

Section I below will shed a different light both on this assumption of piety, and on the aversion to randomness and contingency that underlies theodicy. In suggesting that, on the contrary, there may be something intrinsically sacrilegious about the enterprise, this first section could be said to be doing "meta-theodicy." Section II will then take us beyond the first "aversion" referred to above. That is, it will explore how traditional Jewish texts seriously consider the possibility that contingency and randomness are persistent and pervasive features of the world, even as they affirm the presence of God in that world. It then will fall to Section III to take up the question of how meaningfully motivating and inspiring a divine presence can be in the midst of randomness. This final section thus deals as much with the pastoral aspects of theology as it does with theory.

1. THEODICY: PIETY OR SACRILEGE?

The Torah represents to us repeatedly that catastrophes are connected to sin and punishment.[5] And later, in Rabbinic literature, regarding plague in particular, we find this statement in Mishnah Avot 5:11:

> Pestilence rages in the world at four specific times: in the fourth year [of the sabbatical cycle], and in the seventh year— because of laxity about the rules of the tithes for the poor due in years 3 and 6; at the end of the seventh year—because of laxity regarding the rules of sabbatical year produce; and at the end of the festival of Sukkot in every year—because of the misappropriation of gifts to the poor.

The connection between the outbreak of disease and the commission of sin, and thus the urgency of repentance and scrupulousness in fulfilling religious obligations, is notably persistent and enduring. Throughout the centuries, prayers written for times of plague have most often been *selihot* [penitential prayers]. And, in keeping with a long and continuous tradition in ultra-Orthodox Jewish communities, the current Covid-19

---

[5] Deut. 11 and 28 contain the most comprehensive among such statements.

pandemic has seen the posting of broadsides in those neighborhoods calling for prayer and repentance in order to ameliorate the fury of the plague.

A convenient shorthand for this most conventional of conventional theodicies is "Doing good = Doing well." That is, you will do well (in the sense of prospering) if and only if you do good (in the sense of acting properly).[6]

There are other ways, of course, in which the justification of God has historically been proposed and argued for.[7] They need not be dwelled on here, for even though they follow different strategies, they share the basic characteristic of insisting on the existence of a divine plan that would maximize beneficence for the world.

One may quarrel—even strenuously—with these ways of justifying the ways of God, but how and why might one entertain the idea that there is something *impious* about the enterprise?

This very question is posed by a seemingly counterintuitive scene in a modern work of fiction, Thornton Wilder's Pulitzer Prize-winning novel, *The Bridge of San Luis Rey*. A very sympathetic but misguided character, Brother Juniper, witnesses the catastrophic collapse of a bridge in Peru, which caused five people to fall to their deaths in the deep gorge below. Juniper, motivated by a need to justify the tragedy, decides to devote himself to investigate everything about those five victims in order to clarify why they were brought together at that bridge at that very moment, and why what happened to them was in keeping with a moral economy. He compiles a book of theodicy that strains to argue that both the dead and the survivors had somehow earned their fate. And then, the book comes to the attention of some ecclesiastical judges, and Juniper no doubt expects to be applauded for his faith and for his service of the just God. But instead

---

[6] When the Babylonian Talmud (Tractate Avodah Zarah 17b-18a) tells of the martyrdom of Rabbi Hanina ben Teradyon and his family, it is not satisfied with the simple fact that this was a judgment of a Roman court. There must have been some sin against the God of Israel for this to have occurred, and thus the narrative ends up concocting a trumped-up charge of his having been publicly disrespectful of the ineffable divine name. The Talmudic narrative ends with the condemned Hanina and his kin reciting verses that speak of the unassailable justice of God (verses that are to this day considered part of Jewish liturgy recited at a burial).

[7] For example, Keats' idea that the world is intended by God to be a "vale of soul-making... where the heart must feel and suffer in a thousand diverse ways" in order to be properly schooled. Hyder Edward Rollins, ed., *The Letters of John Keats, 1814-1821* (Cambridge, MA: Harvard University Press, 1958), 100.

the book is condemned by the Church as heretical, and it and poor Brother Juniper are burned in the village square.[8] We are entitled to wonder why.

An initial clue to understanding why such a devotional act aimed at justifying God could be seen as heretical is provided by another detail about Juniper's story. Years earlier, a plague had struck Juniper's own village, and when he studied all that he could about those victims and survivors, he found that the dead seemed to have been five times more worth saving than the survivors. And to this, Wilder laconically adds this quotable line: "The discrepancy between faith and the facts is greater than is generally assumed."[9] That is, attending to *facts* may be as important in the pursuit of God's truth as are our constructed canons of faith.

Wilder wrote a novel, but it is not only in fiction that contriving to explain and thus justify God's ways runs afoul of other pillars of religion. Consider the case of Galileo. What most of us "know"—because so we have been taught—is that Galileo brought the power of the church down on him because he gave credence and support to a view of planetary motion that contradicted the plain meaning of Scripture.

But Wade Rowland, in his book *Galileo's Mistake*, puts forward and documents a different understanding of the conflict. Pope Urban VIII was actually a friend of Galileo's and an admirer and supporter of scientific observation. An apparent contradiction to the plain contextual meaning of Scripture would not, and did not, create a crisis for this man, who was no fool, and an avid follower of scientific discovery. But Urban was threatened by the larger movement into whose ring Galileo had thrown his hat. That was what is known as Mechanism, the idea that there are mechanical laws that are inviolate. It was not "how the heavens go" that irked the theologians who tried Galileo. It was the program to reduce all that happened on earth and in the skies to rigid laws of cause-and-effect. This is what was behind the Pope's complaint that "we should not impose necessity upon the Lord Almighty."[10]

So the Church—not exactly the benighted science-denying gang as

---

[8] Thornton Wilder, *The Bridge of San Luis Rey* (New York: Harper Perennial, 1998), 111.
[9] Wilder, 113.
[10] Wade Rowland, *Galileo's Mistake* (New York: Arcade Publishing, 2001), 239-240.

they are often caricatured—sensed that necessitating God by *physical* laws was an intolerable lèse majesté. In the same way, there is an argument—which at least must be considered—that there may be something theologically awry in necessitating God by *moral* laws that we discern. And that is what *all* theodicies do.

Like Juniper, we imagine that theodicies are meant to serve *God* by saving a sense of divine justice, and thus averting a rejection of the divine because of the all-too-common human experience of apparently gratuitous suffering. But, when all is said and done, they are constructs that *we* create, and we do that in order that we are better able to address and to manage our anxieties, our perplexities, our disappointments, and our anger at the slings and arrows that we suffer. And if they are created to address our fear of that which is random and inexplicable, then they are here to serve *us*, rather than to serve *God*. This is how the common impression that theodicy is a reverent endeavor is undercut.

The biblical book of Job is often thought of as refuting a particular theodicy, namely the "Doing good = Doing well" version. But in fact, Job is one of the most potent arguments against *all* theodicies. Edward Greenstein has lately given us a beautiful new translation of the book with some stunning commentary.[11] Some of what he says in his introduction was already anticipated in the introduction to Job that he wrote for *The Jewish Study Bible*. He starts by noting that everyone who is looking for *the* theodicy ends up frustrated, having read Job:

> There is no resolution to the problem of evil in Job because that is not the theme of the book.... Instead, Job incorporates two main themes. First, the book presents a philosophical argument about how our knowledge is warranted or justified. Job's companions stubbornly cling to the claim that all worthwhile knowledge has been transmitted and learned from tradition.... Job, on the other hand, bases his claims on his personal observation—knowledge can be transformed by new experience, such as what has happened to him[12].... Job's

---

[11] Edward Greenstein, *Job: A New Translation* (New Haven, CT: Yale University Press, 2019).

[12] Greenstein's formulation here is a remarkably faithful echo of the observation made by Stephen Jay Gould that the Renaissance was dedicated to the idea that all knowledge worth

unconventional understanding of God is only confirmed by
the theophany from the 'tempest,' in which the Deity passes
over, and possibly tramples, the principle of just retribution.

A second, and arguably even more prevalent, theme in Job is
that of honesty in talking about God.... [W]hile the friends
regard Job's discourse as no more than hot air... Job takes
pride in his absolute commitment to speaking only truth (Job
27:3-4). The radical turning point in the book comes at its
conclusion: God turns to Job's companions and reproves them
for not speaking "truthfully" about Him as Job "My servant"
had done (42:7-8). Job may not have arrived at the truth, but
he had reason to believe in what he was saying, as it came to
him honestly, unlike the words of the companions, who merely
repeated uncritically the wisdom they had received.[13] Seen this
way, the book of Job promotes honesty in theological discourse
and rejects a blind reliance on tradition.[14]

Note the ire that facile theodicies provoke in God ("I'm incensed at
your friends" as the New JPS renders it).[15] Even as they purport to be pious, the friends are lazy, dishonest, and even slanderous.

And this emphasis on honesty is precisely what Kant was after when
he wrote of the "miscarriage" of all attempts at theodicy.[16]

....[H]onesty in openly admitting one's doubts; repugnance
to pretending conviction where one feels none, especially
before God (where this trick is pointless enough)—these are

---

knowing was inherent in the wisdom of the classical world, whereas the Scientific Revolution insisted that only new observations and discoveries could reliably ground knowledge.
Job's friends reflect the Renaissance ethos, whereas Job represents the scientist who cannot
distrust the experimental evidence. See Stephen Jay Gould, *The Hedgehog, The Fox, and the
Magister's Pox* (New York: Harmony Books, 2003), 36-39.

[13] To use Pope Urban's terminology (though this is surely not the way he would have read
Job), the friends were "necessitating God" by binding God to their received theodicy.

[14] Adele Berlin and Marc Zvi Brettler, eds., *The Jewish Study Bible* (Oxford: Oxford University Press, 2014), 1494.

[15] Job 42:7, in *The Writings* (Philadelphia: Jewish Publication Society of America, 1982)

[16] Kant, 40-41.

the attributes which, in the person of Job, have decided the preeminence of the honest man over the religious flatterer in the divine verdict.... For with this disposition he proved that he did not found his morality on faith, but his faith on morality: in such a case, however weak this faith might be, yet it alone is of a pure and true kind, i.e., the kind of faith that founds not a religion of supplication, but a religion of good life conduct.[17]

For Kant (and for Greenstein's reading of Job), Job's great virtue was not "patience," but rather "truthfulness."

2. THREE SPECIES OF CONTINGENCY

If, as the previous section has argued, theodicy substitutes our preferred conception of God's *modus operandi* for God's absolute freedom, and God is not to be "necessitated" in that way, then we need to investigate whether a religious sense of God's presence can be squared with an acknowledgment of pervasive contingency in the world.

Three texts from the traditional Jewish canon will aid us in this, in that they will be seen to incorporate not only a recognition of contingency in God's world, but an actual *embrace* of it as a foundational truth about the world. The three texts form an ascending sequence in the following way: In the first, we will encounter contingency from our point of view; i.e., all may come from God's will, but since God cannot be necessitated and is unrestrained, that will cannot be predicted, *pace* Job's friends and Brother Juniper. In the second, there is an assertion of contingency that God has ordained, but though having ordained it, God can neither override nor control it. And the third text will present the most pervasive contingency of all, one that is built into the world, entirely independent of God's will.

A. Contingencies owing to our inability to know

In the Babylonian Talmud (Tractate Berakhot 7a) Rabbi Yohanan cites a tradition from Rabbi Yosi that Moses made three requests of God, and all were granted. The third of these was to be informed of God's method

---

[17] This notion of a religion of "good life conduct" will figure below in the theological musings in Section 3.

for meting out prosperity and suffering. After some dead-end speculations about what God told Moses, the best the Talmud can do is to suggest that God's answer is that the righteous who suffer are not "entirely righteous," and the wicked who prosper are not "entirely wicked." But then comes the passage's punchline:

> But all of this is in contradistinction to Rabbi Meir's opinion. For Rabbi Meir said: Two of Moses' requests were granted to him, and one was not granted to him.... God did *not* reveal to Moses the ways in which God conducts the world. As it is said: "And I will be gracious to whom I will be gracious" [Ex. 33:19], even though that person is not worthy. "And I will have mercy upon whom I will have mercy," [ibid.], even though that person is not worthy.

Notice that when the Talmud assumed that God did give Moses an answer to his third request, it struggled to articulate what that answer could possibly have been, and that struggle met contradictions and ultimately ended in the vagueness of "not completely righteous or wicked." But Rabbi Meir, who is elsewhere said to have suffered the sudden and inexplicable death of two young sons, comes forward as the Jobian figure who says "no" to the idea that Moses could have been taught anything about a world in which God cannot be constrained by human needs or even human morality.

So that is contingency from our perspective: God's will is the determinant, but there is no decision procedure by which we can possibly predict what will befall the world and its inhabitants. Covid-19 may come by virtue of the divine will, but not—Rabbi Meir insists—because God wishes us well, and wants us to break our bad habits, change our lives for the better, etc. It is purely because of the freedom of the divine will, having nothing to do with our needs or merits. As Job, the book and the character, puts it (Job 9:12): "Who can say to God, What are You doing?"

B. Contingencies that God has Ordained, and Then Must "Live With"

The next fascinating text moves us away from the idea that God's will is behind every occurrence. It comes from a medieval work by the older contemporary of Maimonides, Abraham ibn Daud. His philosophical work *Ha-emunah ha-Ramah* (known in English as "The Exalted Faith") presents the argument for contingency in this world that is *uncontrolled* by God, because God so *ordained* the world to be.

Here is the relevant passage:

> ".....the 'possible' is of two types:
>
> 'possible' [only] because of our ignorance. ...think about eclipses, and the question of whether one will occur during this month or not. This can only be considered 'possible' by those who are untutored in astronomy; yet one of the two possibilities is surely determined, and God must know which of the two obtains in fact.
>
> But the second type of 'possibility' is this: that the blessed God has decreed that it *be* merely possible. That is, God created things that could bear different attributes that are opposed to each other, as circumstances would have it. In such a case, one ought not recoil from the idea that God knows only the possibilities.
>
> Should one obstinately object that attributing ignorance to God will put us on an untenable path, we answer that this is no ignorance at all. One who insists on this, in reality is attempting to understand every event in the world as one must understand the eclipses—i.e., fully determined. Were that the case, life in this world would be degraded [i.e., a fully determined world would remove all incentive to work and build] and the future world would lose all meaning [for moral merit would become meaningless].[18]

---

[18] Abraham ibn Daud, *Ha-Emunah ha-Ramah*, Hebrew trans. Solomon ben Lavi (Frankfurt, 1852), 96.

That is, certain phenomena and events seem merely contingent (i.e., not necessary) to *us*, because we just don't know enough to make the determination; whereas in and of themselves those events are determined. This second type of possibility is fundamentally different, in that its indeterminism is decreed by God to be so. So we have here randomness, though it is a randomness that is still not separated from God's will, which has ordained it. And that brings us to the third species of contingency, in which the divine will actually recedes.

C. Contingencies in the World that are Entirely Independent of God

This, then, brings us to the most radical of all of the admissions about contingency that we are considering. It is in the Babylonian Talmud (Tractate Hagigah 4b-5a). Rav Beivai bar Abaye witnesses a remarkable scene: The Angel of Death instructs his agent to bring him (i.e., kill) a particular woman, but in a case of mistaken identity, the wrong woman (with the same name) is brought. (She could be snatched because she had a random accident, which weakened her life force.) Rather than return her to life, the Angel of Death decides to keep the unfortunate "impostor." Then the pointed question comes:

> Rav Beivai bar Abaye then said to the Angel of Death: "Have you permission to act in this manner?" The Angel of Death said to him, "And is it not written: 'There are those swept away without justice' (Prov. 13:23)?" Rav Beivai said to him, "But isn't it also written: 'One generation passes away, and another generation comes' (Eccles. 1:4)?" He said to him, "I shepherd them, not releasing them until the years of the generation are completed, and then I pass them on to the angel Duma [who oversees the souls of the dead]."

Note well how ibn Daud emphasizes that contingency is *sine qua non* for the exercise of human moral choice. Maimonides would later attempt to harmonize (in a somewhat tortured way) perfect divine knowledge with human moral agency; ibn Daud takes the simpler approach of denying perfect knowledge to God—a denial ordained by God! We have already seen the connection between contingency and moral life touched on by Kant, and we will visit it again in Section 3 ahead.

And here is David Kraemer's commentary:

> The opinion of this story, in all of its radicalness, is perfectly clear.… The Angel of Death or his messenger can entirely disregard what God's will requires.…
>
> The first and most obvious element of this composition is the complete absence of any explicit mention of God… God is not involved here. God is not an active participant in this death or related matters of justice.…
>
> Moreover, by positing that the death itself is effectuated by an agent of the agent of God, the narrative serves further to symbolically remove this death from God.…
>
> "Have you permission?" is a broad question, and the angel's response makes it clear that he feels he has the overall right to take lives prematurely. If there is any limitation on this power, it is not spelled out. Only an accident is needed before the angel's right is activated, and there can be little question of the prevalence of such accidents.[19]

This third take on contingency—even though in it, God is so absent—is, I want to argue, the most promising way of reacting theologically to pandemics and to so many more catastrophic occurrences. Suggesting such a theological direction is now the subject of the next, and last, section.

3. IS THERE A WORKABLE THEOLOGY IN ALL THIS?

What has made the "Doing good = Doing well" theodicy as agreeable, and thus as persistent, as it has been is this: When people are told that it is their sins that had perforce, and inevitably, brought on their woes, they now have a roadmap for how to reverse their ill fortune. Randomness

---

[19] David Kraemer, *Responses to Suffering in Classical Rabbinic Literature* (Oxford: Oxford University Press, 1995), 203-204.

can break a sense of continuity, apparently revealing it to be an illusion, one that can be shattered by whatever accidental event next comes along. Contrition for sins, on the other hand, reveals instead a *continuity* of covenant that one can count on.

But if we are to accept a ubiquitous contingency, will we be able to refashion a world of faith, and of moral action, given experiences such as pandemics? This question presses upon us at moments such as this, when random mutations and chance encounters between different species (in a faraway wet market) can create mass suffering and death in our world.[20] Is there a way of speaking of God that makes sense intellectually and spiritually—and, crucially, that has ethical integrity—as we come to grips with the unremitting contingency of events on this earth?

In a secular context that nevertheless is relevant here, Richard Rorty has argued that if we accept that contingency is pervasive in the world, then the idea that there is a conscious master plan antecedent to the world cannot stand:

> In his Dewey Lectures, [John] Rawls echoes both [Isaiah] Berlin and Dewey when he says:
>
> What justifies a conception of justice is not its being true to an order antecedent and given to us, but its congruence with our deeper understanding of ourselves and our aspirations, and our realization that, given our history and the traditions embedded in our public life, it is the most reasonable doctrine for us.
>
> ... [This] way of looking at morality as a set of practices, our practices, makes vivid the difference between the conception of morality as the voice of a divinized portion of our soul, and as the voice of a contingent human artifact, a community which has grown up subject to the vicissitudes of time and chance, one more of Nature's "experiments."[21]

---

[20] The front page of the July 1, 2020 print edition of the New York Times featured an article about a New Jersey family upon which the current pandemic had inflicted Jobian-level tragedies: The family's 73-year-old matriarch, three of her 11 children, and her sister all died of Covid-19.

[21] Richard Rorty, *Contingency, Irony, and Solidarity* (Cambridge: Cambridge University

That is, we have to build our world and our convictions out of experience, just as Job had learned, and not out of an *a priori* narrative, as his friends had insisted. There may be no conscious master plan that explains the Jobian agony of the sufferers of today—and of all yesterdays (see Note 11 for one poignant current example of such agony). So what do we think and do now?

Well, what did Job finally do? There is not universal agreement on the meaning of what Job says after the Whirlwind Speech has ended (see Job 42:2-6). But there are strong reasons to prefer one of them to all the others. Conventionally, 42:6 is considered to be part of Job's "recantation." It is, for example, rendered by the Revised Standard Version as "therefore I despise myself, and repent in dust and ashes."[22] But why would Job retract all that he had said between chapters 3 and 31? Because of the Speech from the Whirlwind, which, for all its poetic grandeur, utterly fails to address Job's pain and complaint?

Here is what Jack Miles has to say, in his ambitious work detailing the biography of God as presented in the Hebrew Bible:

> We come now to the linchpin of the traditional interpretation, the cryptic closing verse of Job's speech.... in the RSV translation:
>
> *Therefore I despise myself, and repent in dust and ashes.*[23]
>
> This is the filament from which hangs the thread from which hangs the entire traditional reading of Job's last words as a recantation. If the first four verses in the speech have usually been translated to read as a recantation, it is because they have all been interpreted in the light of this closing verse. In the Hebrew, however, this verse is ambiguous, and in the RSV's resolution of the ambiguity no word has less support from the original than the word "myself." ... Against the traditional interpretation, it is likely that though Job is in the grip of

---

Press, 1989), 58-60.

[22] The New JPS translation has "therefore, I recant and relent, being but dust and ashes."

[23] Jack Miles, *God: A Biography* (New York: Vintage Books, 1995), 323-325.

profoundly changed and negative feelings about something at this point, that something is not himself.

Job was concerned, of course, about the implications for his fellow men should God prove to be what he seemed to be for Job. Reading "dust and ashes" as an expression of this concern, as a reference to mankind in its mortal frailty, reading the verbs that the RSV translates "despise myself, and repent" as transitive, with "dust and ashes" or (more idiomatically) "mortal clay" as their common object, we may translate the closing words:

Now that my eyes have seen you,
I shudder with sorrow for mortal clay.

Or, as Greenstein renders it:

That is why I am fed up; I take pity on dust and ashes.[24]

Far from a penitential recanting, in this rendering—which is much more consistent with all that we have seen of Job for the previous 39 chapters—Job recognizes the capricious and thus meaningless contingency that has crushed him, and, in disgust at the random meaninglessness of his suffering, he resigns the case that he had thought to prosecute when he supposed that God is somehow bound to follow the contours of a humanly composed theodicy.

And yet, the book does not end there. Along comes an epilogue, in which God says something wholly unexpected. Here it is in the new Greenstein translation:

It happened, after YHWH spoke these words to Job, that YHWH said to Eliphaz the Teimanite: I am angry at you and your two companions, for you did not speak about me in honesty as did my servant Job. Now then, take yourselves seven bulls and seven rams and go to my servant Job, and offer up

---

[24] Greenstein, 185

a burnt-offering on your own behalf; and my servant Job will pray for you; for I will lift up his face without doing anything unseemly to you—for you did not speak about me in honesty as did my servant Job.[25]

What has happened here, and how and why might it have affected Job? In particular, what prompts this admission from God that it was Job, all along, who spoke the truth in this book?

Carl Gustav Jung gave his understanding of God's recantation (if we can call it that) in his book entitled *Answer to Job*, in which the "answer" proposed is the Christian belief known as the Incarnation. He proposes an explanation for what it was—when the human psyche attempted to channel the divine psyche—that gave rise to the idea that God had to become a human being:

> God does not want to be just; he merely flaunts might over right. Job could not get that into his head, because he looked upon God as a moral being. He had never doubted God's might, but had hoped for right as well.... [God's] thunderings at Job so completely miss the point that one cannot help but see how much he is occupied with himself....

> The victory of the vanquished and oppressed is obvious: Job stands morally higher than Yahweh. In this respect the creature has surpassed the creator. Job's superiority cannot be shrugged off.... and thus makes possible Y ahweh's decision to become man.... he raises himself above his earlier primitive level of consciousness by indirectly acknowledging that the man Job is morally superior to him and that therefore he has to catch up and become human himself. Had he not taken this decision he would have found himself in flagrant opposition to his omniscience.[26]

---

[25] Greenstein, 186-187.

[26] C.G. Jung, *Answer to Job*, trans. R.F.C. Hull (Princeton, NJ: Princeton University Press, 1969), 16, 42-43.

You can think of this as a commentary on the brief Epilogue to Job. After all, what *would* the author of Job imagine God being moved to say after the Whirlwind Speech, and after Job's expression of nothing but pity for mortal humans buffeted by the whims of an amoral God? When what has been exposed is the yawning gap between the morally thinking and sensitive human, who demands right, and the Godly, creative Force behind it all, which does not—because it *cannot*—speak of right, but only of might.

The non sequitur character of the Whirlwind Speech only makes sense if God is, in fact, utterly incapable of understanding Job's demand for justice. Which means that, despite what Genesis 1 told us, we are not actually made in the image of God, because we are radically unlike. From Genesis 1 right through the Torah, the Prophets, and the first three books of the Writings, we have carried with us this idea that we are God-like, and that God is in significant ways like us. But the truth-teller has now corrected that comforting but incorrect idea. And that truth-teller, we now know, is Job, who is (to advert to Gould's prototypes—see Note 12) not the Renaissance man, but the experimental and experiential scientist.

This prepares us for what Jack Miles matter-of-factly reveals to us:

> A view common to nearly all commentators on the Book of Job is that, one way or another, the Lord has reduced Job to virtual silence. Unnoticed is the fact that from the end of the Book of Job to the end of the Tanakh, God never speaks again.[27]

And what now happens to Job? Apparently he is now—as opposed to just a few verses earlier—no longer resigned in disgust to the inevitable blows that the world by contingent chance inflicts on all without moral discrimination. He faces not a personal, active, capricious God, but rather a God for whom the moral truth that matters so much to Job is not really recognizable; not because of malevolence, *but because God is utterly different*. In the aftermath of the Whirlwind Speech, Job was like Rabbi Meir of Berakhot, who believed that God had a plan, but was resigned to an inability to scrutinize the divine ways. Now, after God's admission that Job has a truth that escapes even God, Job's position is more like that which Kraemer explicated in the Hagigah text—living in a world of accidents in

---

[27] Miles, 329

which God is not implicated, and from which God is quite removed. No longer wallowing in perpetual disgust, he forgives his friends and makes offerings for them. He prays for them. And while we know him to have been smart enough never to have entirely given up mourning his losses, he was able to come to terms with life, and even enjoy what it brought him in his many later years. For that's how the book finally ends, not with a Job saying *I am fed up*, but instead "old and sated with days."

It seems that a theological revelation that is so jarring to the traditional tropes has somehow bestowed a sober and very humane equanimity on the sorely injured, but not chastened, Job.

So what about this God—who does not reside on the plane of moral reasoning, yet whose presence no longer terrifies and disgusts Job? If we were to throw at this God the questions we ask ourselves in the last hour of Yom Kippur (What are we? What is the meaning of our existence? Our power? Our goodness?),[28] what would God's answers be?

For this, I offer just one possibility, from the theological case that Arthur Green puts forth in *Radical Judaism*:

> The entire course of evolution, from the simplest life forms millions of years ago, to the great complexity of the human brain (still now only barely understood), and proceeding onward into the unknown future, [I take] to be a *meaningful* process. There is a One that is ever revealing itself to us within and behind the great diversity of life. That One is Being itself, the constant in the endlessly changing evolutionary parade....
>
> That has caused it to bring about, in the long and slow course of its evolution, the emergence of a mind that can reflect upon the process, articulate it, and strive toward the life of complete awareness that will fulfill its purpose....
>
> The descendants of one-celled creatures grew and developed, emerged onto dry land, learned survival skills, developed language and thought, until a subset of them could reflect on

---

[28] These are questions that appear prominently in the final "Ne'ilah" service on the Day of Atonement.

the nature of this entire process and seek to derive meaning from it.[29]

What makes this understanding of God particularly apt as we ponder the ineluctable randomness in the world is that *randomness is precisely the mechanism by which evolution proceeds* and, in this vision, by which the divine reveals itself. If we began thinking that randomness challenged theology, then this is one of the antidotes to such thoughts. And in this conception of things, we humans who have evolved a moral and ethical sense—not to mention awesome intellectual and scientific prowess—are not *surpassers* of the Creator, as Jung put it, but rather *fulfillers* of the power of the Creator. There is *hesed*—mercy, pity—in God, but not as a grant from beyond us, but rather in what of God we have revealed, by having evolved by the ultimate power of God, Being, the One.

Contingency will always be with us. Human evil will be with us. But so, inevitably, will tsunamis, asteroid strikes that extinguish species, and sadly, Covid-19 as well. That plenitude of possibility is the answer to "What is God's power?" And the answer to "What is God's goodness?" is: The manifestation of God's power in the human being is where goodness resides. The gifts of moral sense and compassion can bring us meaning, even as we are forced to give up on the sincere, but misguided, quest for a theodicy.[30]

Isn't it fascinating, to continue Miles' train of thought about God's final words in the Hebrew Bible, that when we turn the page after completing the very heavy book of Job, the very next page brings us to the Song of Songs, and the pleasure that the plenitude of God's world brings to us? And the capacity for compassion that the awesome power of creation as the unfolding of God's power has given us? Perhaps that's why Thornton Wilder ended his novel with these words:

---

[29] Arthur Green, *Radical Judaism: Rethinking God and Tradition* (New Haven, CT: Yale University Press, 2010), 20-21

[30] Two Finnish philosophers, Sari Kivistö and Sami Pihlström have articulated, in Kantian style, this central ethical element of a theology of contingency: "The falsity of the friends' views also stems from their intellectual efforts to construct tenable narratives in order to explain Job's turmoil, and thus their mistake has a moral basis. Especially after the Second World War….instead of building explanations and appealing to fictive causation [we] should aim to relieve misery by helping the victims." Sari Kivistö and Sami Pihlström, "Kantian Anti-Theodicy and Job's Sincerity," Philosophy and Literature 40, no. 2 (2016): 356-358.

There is a land of the living and a land of the dead
and the bridge is love, the only survival, the only meaning.

Loving God Through Life and Death:
An Embodied Theology of Loss

Aviva Richman

One central challenge in a time of intense loss and tragedy is how to translate divine love into terms that are comprehensible. Pain is usually seen as a theological obstacle, and many approaches to theology and suffering have emerged over time, aiming to reconcile divine love and loss. From talmudic sages after the destruction of the Temple to post-Holocaust theologians, the Jewish tradition has struggled with what it means to be in relationship with God in a world where God feels decidedly absent. Living through plague exacerbates the already existing problem. Where is God when hundreds of thousands of people are dying? The amount of ink spilled on these questions over the centuries is indication enough that there are no satisfying answers. But this does not mean that all of the unsatisfying answers are the same; there is a lot at stake in how we approach questions of suffering and theodicy. Where are *we* when we try to locate God in suffering and loss? What is asked of us and how do we conceive of our own capacities as we try to gain a better sense of where God is?

One response articulated in classical rabbinic sources, recapitulated and developed into modernity, is the notion that God's presence in the world manifests in our own realization of our divine capacity, *tzelem Elohim*. We are created in God's image not in any sort of physical way but by virtue of imitating God, by walking in God's ways.[1] Walking in God's ways can be understood as an act of mirroring what God already does, but it can mean something more radical against a backdrop of our sense of divine absence. Staring into the void, we come to realize that our own actions have the power to bring God into the world. If we are meant to imitate God and visit the sick, but we live in a world where we see that the sick are abandoned, then when we visit the sick we are the agents who bring the divine presence into the world. Our own human potential—and

---

[1] For some foundational sources on the idea of walking in God's ways, see Deuteronomy 28:9, Sifre Deuteronomy Eikev 11:22, and Maimonides Mishneh Torah Deot 1:5.

responsibility—take center stage in the work of *Imitatio Dei*—striving to walk in God's ways.

Yet, even as it can amplify human agency, *Imitatio Dei* is clearly a constrained exercise, subject to our own inadequacies and failings as mere mortals. There are boundaries of how far finite beings can go to do the work of the Infinite. Clearly, we are not all-knowing, nor all-just, nor all-powerful. We cannot bring people back to life. We cannot end a plague. What is meant, then, to be the scope of *Imitatio Dei*? In what ways, exactly, can we become like God, and how might our sense of the God we are trying to imitate and our sense of our capacity to imitate shift in times of plague?

This essay traces a pathway towards approaching loss not as a thorny theodicy obstacle, but rather—in a mode of radical acceptance—to understand our encounter with loss as one dimension of how we might be able to be like God. In the wake of widespread death and loss, we may need to be ready to imitate God in new ways.

Imitatio Dei I: Our Divine Capacity to do Hesed

One dominant strain of the concept of *Imitatio Dei* suggests that being like God specifically relates to our capacity to do *hesed* (lovingkindness). The earliest articulation of this idea is found in a third century midrash:

> זה אלי ואנוהו...אבא שאול אומר אדמה לו מה הוא רחום וחנון אף אתה רחום וחנון.

> This is my God and I will glorify [God]" (Exodus 15:2)...
> Abba Shaul says: I will be like God. Just as God is merciful and gracious, so you should be merciful and gracious.
> —*Mekhilta d'Rabbi Yishmael,* The Song #3

Abba Shaul here delineates an approach of "becoming like" the divine, but not in all ways. He enumerates only God's attributes of mercy and compassion. He does not mention God's attributes of justice, or anger, or jealousy. The Babylonian Talmud (Sotah 14a) records a more detailed and practical version of this tradition, where the way we follow in God's ways is to clothe the naked, visit the sick, comfort mourners, and bury the dead. Highlighting God's care-work aligns, albeit selectively, with attributes of God listed in Psalm 146, where God redresses injustice against the downtrodden, gives food to the hungry, frees those who are bound, and protects strangers, orphans, and widows.

A straightforward reading of the classical midrash suggests that God *already does* all of these deeds of lovingkindness—one might even say that they are God's signature—and our role is to do our best, in our limited capacity, to try to imitate God's infinite capacity for kindness. A more recent reading of these texts developed by R. Yitzhak Hutner (1906-1980) offers a more radical reading of *Imitatio Dei*. In the opening essay of his series devoted to *hesed* at the beginning of his writings on the holiday of Rosh Hashanah, R. Hutner paints a picture in which God cannot exist in our world if we do not engage in *hesed*. God's presence is *contingent on* our acts of *hesed*, so to speak. The starkest formulation of his approach is that God does not reign—God is essentially absent from our world—if *we* do not initiate God-like activities of compassion and kindness in our world.

> For just as without the Creator's attribute of *hesed*, as it were, there is no place for created beings, so too without the attribute of *hesed* of those created beings there is no place for the Creator, as it were...[2]

When we see a lack of God's presence in the world, the next move is not to point our finger in blame at God, with sharp critiques of God's negligence. The next move is to point a finger at ourselves and ask what kindness we can do, to activate the potential for divine presence in our world.

This beautiful reading can go far in a state of plague. Certainly the divine roles of tending to the sick, comforting mourners, and burying the dead require profound attention and manifold repetition in our moment. Naming this work as divine work hopefully calls greater attention to all of those who engage in this difficult, sometimes tedious, and rather uncomfortable labor, and greatly elevates the value of their work.

But in a time of plague, this capacity to imitate God is not enough. As beautiful an idea as it may be, it does not fully respond to the scale of loss

---

[2] R. Yitzhak Hutner. *Kuntres ha-Hesed Collection of Essays on Hesed*, #1.

we see and feel in these times. We cannot stop at Abba Shaul's succinct, if profound, charge to cling to God's ways only by being merciful and gracious. There is another capacity of God that we can, and must, strive to embody.

Imitatio Dei II: Our Divine Capacity to Hold Death and Loss

The actions that represent God's capacity for *hesed* do not only appear in the literary traditions of Bible, Midrash, and philosophy; they are also ritualized liturgically as a central motif in daily prayer. The second blessing of the *Amidah*, *Gevurot* (God's strengths), includes some of the list of God's attributes from Psalm 146, along with other acts of kindness, integrated under the heading that God "sustains life with *hesed*." We might easily read this list as strengths that distinguish the divine capacity from anything within human reach. Indeed, it includes praise for God "who brings the dead to life." Yet based on what we learned above it seems that we actually are meant to strive to emulate even life-giving.

This second blessing includes not only the life-giving capacity of God (*mehayeh*) but also the capacity of death (*memit*). The line between life and death is so very fragile and mysterious that it is often perceived to be the quintessence of God's domain, beyond human control. One might therefore conclude that while the life-giving parts of this blessing do fall under the charge of *Imitatio Dei*, the death-dealing ones do not.

I would like to suggest the contrary; that especially in the midst of plague, our human capacity to imitate the divine capacity to hold death can, and perhaps must, be exercised as part of the fullness of our *tzelem Elohim*. To demonstrate what this means, let us turn to another passage in R. Hutner's essays.

In a discussion of ways of loving God, R. Hutner references the first paragraph of the *Shema*: "You shall love your God with all of your heart, with all of your might and with all of your soul" (Deuteronomy 6:5). Drawing on the Talmud's interpretation of these three pathways in Mishnah Brachot 9:5 (heart, might, and soul), R. Hutner focuses on the word "one" (*ehad*) at the end of the first sentence of *Shema*, and suggests that all of these ways of loving God are essentially about the work of integration; all involve synthesizing two apparent binaries. God's one-ness means that if we are created in God's image, we also must strive for one-ness. Part of our work, then, in walking in God's ways is to create harmony between apparent binaries:

> We find that the unity of the Blessed One is revealed in integrating binaries into one entity. Since the obligation is cast upon us to become similar to God, as it were, according to our capacity, the question arises—in what way can we find the capacity to be like God in the description of unity?

> As an answer to this question the words of the sages come to teach us the interpretation of the verse "You shall love Hashem your God." Did not the sages say this in their explanation of this verse:

> "With all of your heart—with your two inclinations"—that is, integrating the binary of the "bad inclination" and "good inclination" to one entity.

> "With all your soul—even if [God] takes your soul"—that is to say, integrating the binary of the realms of death and life to one entity.

> "With all your might—with whatever measure [God] measures out for you"—that is to say, integrating the binaries of the general attributes to one entity.

> Any listening ear will hear and discern a voice breaking through these three interpretations given by the sages for heart, soul, and might, mentioned in the Torah, for the common denominator in these explanations is that they establish the entire stature of a person on profound spiritual unity... The intent of these three interpretations is to teach about the similarity of the created to the Creator in terms of the attribute of unity...[3]

---

[3] R. Yitzhak Hutner, Shavuot Essay #23

While this discussion is quite complex, I will focus here on the italicized section, where loving God with all of our soul somehow requires finding an integration between life and death. What does this aspect of imitating God mean when contextualized within the other, more dominant, approach to imitating God by emulating God's *hesed*?

These two comments of R. Hutner, when read side by side and when taken alongside the second blessing of the Amidah that articulates the divine attribute of sustaining life—and death—through *hesed*, suggest that our work in developing our divine capacity has to include how we approach death and loss. Our mortal world includes death, though many of us in the western world manage to avoid encountering it. We seal it off in contained and mostly invisible places. We "bury" death, literally and figuratively, wanting it to be invisible and far away. There is a class of professionals who do the dirty work of encountering death more closely, but mostly it is God who holds the dead, in the earth, out of our sight. In a time of plague, however, the fact of death as part of our world becomes inescapably visible. We are called to be ready to exercise not only the life-giving divine work of *hesed*, but also the divine work of *hesed* that acknowledges and accompanies death.

Imitatio Dei III: An Embodied Approach to Holding Loss

What enables each of us to be able to exercise this divine capacity to hold loss? There may be myriad experiences we each draw upon. I would like to highlight one embodied form of this capacity for loss that is often culturally invisible, and has in many ways been radically shifted by contemporary medical science.

The Talmud offers many names for female reproductive anatomy. One name for the uterus is *kever*—a grave (e.g., b. Niddah 21a). This reflects a sad, but real, aspect of human reproduction; in the case of pregnancy loss the womb turns into a container for the dead, much like the earth in a graveyard. The idea of the uterus as a grave becomes all the more profound, though, when we realize that before the advent of ultrasounds, people would not automatically know that a pregnancy had been lost, and they could have carried a lost pregnancy for many months before miscarriage or stillbirth. The miscarriages that quickly lead to procedures to remove the fetus nowadays, for the sake of preventing any harm to a mother's body, would have lingered much longer. In other words, much more often pregnancy would have involved uncertainty about whether one's womb was functioning as a cradle for life or a home for death. The human body participated more fully in the work that is now done primarily by the earth, acting as a receptacle that holds death—death that is an inevitable aspect of a world of human life.

I bring this example as someone who carried a twin pregnancy, knowing for months that one fetus had been lost but needing to hold it inside to carry the other fetus to term. For four months I was a *kever*, a walking graveyard, so to speak, and inasmuch as this was hard and sad, it was also a window into an experience that used to be much more common. It was also a profound experience that forced me into a different standpoint relative to loss. I learned that the human body's capacity to hold loss alongside life participates in the divine work of holding both. Even as it was so hard, it also felt like actualizing a capacity of God's role in the world to be able to be close to death. Though I never imagined this was something I would or could do, when I had to do it I suddenly felt much more aware of all of the ways we tend to hide loss, relegating it out of sight to God's realm. Knowing so tangibly that having the capacity to produce life sits right next to the capacity to hold death gave me a new sense of the integration of these divine roles.

A feminist reading of the second blessing of the *Amidah,* wherein God both gives both life and death, alongside R. Hutner's approach to the unifying work of *Imitatio Dei,* leads to a concrete understanding of how we too might hold life and death. How might we recognize and exercise our own God-like capacity to synthesize? We might hold loss literally in our own bodies, as I did, but this example is meant to represent a capacity that extends to various aspects of our psychological and spiritual beings. Holding loss could mean being aware each day of the many people dying in a plague, and carrying that with us in every moment, not in a way that shuts down our capacity to live, but can sit alongside it. Holding loss could mean fully articulating what we have already lost in chaotic circumstances and naming our fears of what we might yet lose, in a way that sharpens, rather than shuts down, our capacity to hope and dream.

Though the quality and scope of our capacity to hold loss is of an entirely different nature than that which we ascribe to God, walking in God's ways involves a willingness to engage with and stretch our own capacities to confront loss.

Conclusion

What it means to be in relationship with God, and even to love God, in a time of plague is not simply an intellectual exercise shaped by intricate philosophical debates about theodicy and the problem of suffering. We will never be able to describe fully who God is or where God is in times like these. Instead, or in parallel, the charge to "walk in God's ways" asks us *who we are* in times like these, and what we need to activate in ourselves in order to bring into being the God we want to see in the world. Much of this path resides in profoundly important and far-reaching care work, which is nothing less than an instantiation of divine *hesed* that sustains the world day in and day out. We are and will continue to be stretched to the limits of our capacity to do care work; but our capacity for *hesed* is not adequate to face the challenge of plague. When we are overwhelmed by loss, rather than bury it out of sight, we can be challenged and comforted to know that part of what it means to actualize our divine potential, our *tzelem Elohim*, is to participate in the divine work of holding death alongside the life that remains.

The Natural Disaster Theology Dilemma

David Zvi Kalman

"When they shake, the world shakes."

This is what the *rosh yeshiva* (head) of my high school said in front of the entire student body on December 27, 2004, the morning after a massive earthquake off the Indonesian coast erupted in a series of deadly tsunamis. The earthquake, the third largest ever recorded, ultimately killed almost a quarter of a million people. The shaking that he was referring to was sex between men, an activity which the Jerusalem Talmud vividly describes as a cause of earthquakes. Says Rav Aha:

> So says the Holy Blessed One: you shake your member over that which is not yours? I shall surely shake my world because of that man.[1]

Tit for tat, shake for shake. In this Talmudic passage, this description of gay sex is only the most striking of several explanations given for fatal natural disasters. But regardless of the specific explanation, it is clear that the rabbis were fully on board with the idea that perceived moral lapses might lead God to wreak havoc on entire populations. In this, the rabbis had strong precedent. Not a few Biblical stories—Noah and the flood, Sodom and Gomorrah, Jonah and Nineveh, the plagues in Egypt, among others—allow that God is ready and willing to bring the forces of nature to bear against the masses as punishment for failing to follow God's rules. This destruction is just one of the manifestations of the concept of reward and punishment that is plastered across the Bible.

This divine characteristic is not something marginal. In Judaism, as in so many religions in antiquity, the divine ability to wield weather patterns in response to human actions is an edifice of faith. The second paragraph of the *Shema* for example, makes a direct connection between human activity and the success of crops:

---

[1] y. Berakhot 9:2 (64a)

If you obey the commandments that I charge you with today...I will grant rain for your land in season, the early rain and the late...Be careful not to be lured away to serve other gods and bow to them, for God's anger will flare up against you, and God will shut up the skies so that there will be no rain and the ground with not yield its produce.[2]

In some ancient religions, questioning this power would have been tantamount to expressing disbelief in the divinity itself, or at least exceeding the bounds of religious discourse. Indeed, Aristotle considered Thales of Miletus (ca. 624–546 BCE) to be the very first philosopher precisely because he was the first to posit that natural phenomena, including earthquakes and weather events, were governed by a principle other than the will of the gods (namely, water).[3]

Despite the strength of the tradition on this point, many moderns, even those who identify themselves as believers, are reticent to ascribe to God these responsibilities. While it is one thing to say that our actions have divine consequences, it is quite another to say that *this* action had *that* consequence, that God sealed the fate of a quarter of a million people, a third of whom were children, because somewhere—along the Thai coast? Throughout Indonesia? Across Southeast Asia?—gay sex was just getting out of hand.

Many people were shaken by my *rosh yeshiva*'s comments that day. Blaming a person for their own death is always a delicate matter, even if all agree that the deceased was not blameless; even a lifelong smoker who dies of lung cancer is not castigated graveside. But a tsunami victim really is blameless in their own demise; to fault such a person for their death is not just impolite, but a diminishment of the deceased's value as a human being. If God kills a person because someone *else* was having gay sex, the victim's life—not to mention their possible virtue—must not have meant very much at all. Ironically, then, it is exactly those circumstances classified as "acts of God" where stipulating that God acted seems most offensive.

---

[2] Deut. 11:13–17. (NJPS translation, modified)
[3] Aëtius, Placita, I.3 and III.15. See also Jaap Mansfeld, "Aristotle and Others on Thales, or the Beginnings of Natural Philosophy," Mnemosyne 38, no. 1–2 (1985): 109–29.

But this is where things get tricky. It turns out that this theology, simultaneously ineffable, deeply-sourced, and blasphemous, is structurally identical to the very critiques that are regularly leveled against governments and corporations in the wake of natural disasters. Perhaps we do not believe that innocent people died because of homosexual activity—but we do believe that they died because a corporation built its nuclear power plant too close to the sea, one reason why Japan's Fukushima Daiichi plant experienced a partial meltdown after a 2011 tsunami. Perhaps we do not agree with televangelist Pat Robertson that the 2010 earthquake in Haiti, which killed one hundred thousand people, was caused because the country's founders "got together and swore a pact to the devil"[4]—but we know that many lives would have been saved had the government prevented builders from using cheap and weak concrete in construction.[5] Perhaps we do not believe that the novel coronavirus, which at the time of writing has killed more than 500,000 people in America alone, is a divine punishment—but many do believe that better government policies could have prevented many of those deaths. We do not actually oppose assigning blame for the deaths of the innocent on the moral failings of others. We just take offense when the connection seems implausible.

Three Faults in Natural Disaster Theology

Because everything hinges on plausibility, blame for the havoc wreaked by natural disasters can reach with ease into both theodicy and politics, often at the same time. This blame game represents a unique entanglement of divine and human responsibility in which both God and humans can and are cited as causal explanations for the same devastating event. Unfortunately, this blame game plays out in exactly those devastating circumstances where people are most desperate to find meaning and most open to changing behaviors. I wish to argue that this entanglement is corrosive to theology. There are three reasons for this, one theological and two political.

First, this entanglement is uniquely theologically fraught, because it

---

[4] "Pat Robertson Says Haiti Paying for 'Pact to the Devil,'" CNN.Com, January 13, 2010.

[5] Joel F. Audefroy, "Haiti: Post-Earthquake Lessons Learned from Traditional Construction," Environment and Urbanization 23, no. 2 (October 10, 2011): 447–62, https://doi.org/10.1177/0956247811418736.

forces a choice between four options that, for moderns, range from unsatisfying to offensive. The first option is to affirm that God is responsible but basically inscrutable, a solution that nominally resolves the entanglement problem by calling it unanswerable, but closes off all further theological discussion in the process.[6] Second, we can claim that God is responsible, but is only acting to punish sinners (the "shakers"). This is problematic for the reasons described above. Third, we can follow the path established within Christian theology by Open Theists and claim that God's providence and/or omnipotence do not preclude the inherent chaos of the universe, and so disasters are literally no one's fault.[7] Finally, we can pass the buck by claiming that God's activity does not exclude the possibility of human error and malice—thereby excusing God, but also excising any hope of extracting deeper meaning from an experience of deep loss.

Compounding these impoverished options is the fact that they are typically deployed in ways that incline people to discount them as facetious. Politicians or corporations which respond to natural disasters by shrugging their shoulders and pointing a finger at God, or at the unpredictability of the natural world, are usually not making serious or sophisticated theological claims, but simply shifting the focus away from themselves. A useful example: the phrase "act of God" was only introduced into English common law in the seventeenth century as a mechanism by which individuals could be absolved of responsibility for damage. It was never intended as a serious theological claim; "God" here has no theological meaning at all, only a legal one.[8] To put this another way: natural disasters have a way of making theologians out of politicians and politicians out of theologians. Such explanations, built to obscure liability rather than help us make sense of a broken world, are rightly regarded with suspicion.

Finally, natural disasters are not just susceptible to weak theologies, offensive theologies, and opportunistic theologies. Most dangerous of all, they are also susceptible to theologically-informed public policy, which is often designed to allow ill effects by perceived "sinners" to continue in

---

[6] This we might think of as the "God in the whirlwind" response, since it resembles God's non-answer to Job about why the latter experienced so much suffering (Job 38:1–18). See Gordon Tucker's essay in this volume for a treatment of this Jobian trope.

[7] For an overview of this movement as it relates to weather, see Peter J. Thuesen, *Tornado God: American Religion and Violent Weather* (Oxford University Press, 2020), 152–156.

[8] Thuesen, 67.

order to reinforce an existing belief that God punishes bad deeds. These policies have a long history of clashing with scientific advances. Anesthesia during childbirth, for example, was panned in its early days on the rationale—sometimes stated explicitly, sometimes not—that birth pains are a curse imposed on women by God after the Fall (Gen. 3:16).[9] At one time, similar logic motivated resistance to the installation of lightning rods, which channel lightning safely away from buildings, on the argument that people should not stop God from destroying buildings as a sign of wrath, especially the tall, prominent ones that seemed to get hit most often.[10]

Even in places where policies are no longer being described in such nakedly theological terms, the same ill effects can still manifest. In the United States, such policies are closely associated with the AIDS epidemic. Though not all early AIDS deaths could be linked to sex between men, the early observed connection between this activity and the sickness initially called "gay-related immune deficiency" (GRID) caused the Reagan administration to speak of the disease in hushed tones while the virus spread, likely slowing the development of effective treatments. Preventative strategies, too, were shaped by Christian morality. Rather than increase funding for sex education or promote the use of condoms, the CDC instead focused its public messaging on abstinence and the closure of bathhouses.[11] When a government responds to a disaster by ignoring science, it runs the risk of causing greater harm in the short term and leaves the door open to further disasters down the road. To make decisions in this manner today, when science and technology allow us to identify effective protective measures, is perhaps the most dangerous possible consequence of entanglement.

---

[9] Carolyn Corretti and Sukumar P. Desai, "The Legacy of Eve's Curse: Religion, Childbirth Pain, and the Rise of Anesthesia in Europe: C. 1200-1800s," Journal of Anesthesia History 4, no. 3 (July 2018): 187–188, https://doi.org/10.1016/j.janh.2018.03.009.

[10] On the lightning rod controversy, see, for example, Eleanor M. Tilton, "Lightning-Rods and the Earthquake of 1755," New England Quarterly 13, no. 1 (1940): 85–97.

[11] Anthony M. Petro, After the Wrath of God: AIDS, Sexuality, and American Religion (Oxford University Press, 2015), chapter 2.

A Theological Growth Area

At best, natural disaster theologies are feeble; at worst, they are deadly. But whether benign or malignant, such theologies present themselves today as a foreign mass, ideologically unwanted and regarded with suspicion because of its potential to kill the host. Perhaps it is best to treat this arm by cutting it off. Though he would not have put it in those words, this seems to have been the approach of Rabbi Lord Immanuel Jakobovits (1921-1999) who, in the midst of the AIDS epidemic, cautioned anyone from casting blame on any individual, saying that no good will ever again come from Jews looking for divine answers to questions of mass suffering. "In the immediate aftermath of the Holocaust," he wrote, "where millions of Jews were done to death with the most unspeakable brutality. We certainly should beware of ever identifying specific forms of grief, suffering, or anxiety with specific moral or any other shortcomings."[12]

For Jakobovits, theological conversations about natural disasters are non-starters—and perhaps, if mass casualty events were few and far between, this radical theological surgery would be enough. But this is not the case. Instead, natural disaster theology and its associated divine/human entanglements are becoming increasingly ubiquitous in the public consciousness, pushing this theological question from the periphery to the center. This is happening for two reasons.

The first reason is that human industry and innovation have created a world in which virtually all of the items traditionally (and even Biblically) associated with God can now plausibly be blamed on people. Famine is the most important example of this phenomenon. As Amartya Sen argued almost 40 years ago, modern famines are no longer the result of poor weather, but instead sprout almost exclusively from poor policy.[13] Other acts of God have plausible human culpability, too. We don't cause major earthquakes (although fracking does cause minor ones), but we can mitigate their effects, both before and after the fact, if we so choose. We don't cause hurricanes or start all wildfires, but human-caused climate change makes each worse. The novel coronavirus was not manufactured

---

[12] Gad Freudenthal, ed., *AIDS in Jewish Thought and Law* (Brooklyn: Ktav, 1998), 11–22.

[13] Amartya Sen, *Poverty and Famine: An Essay on Entitlement and Deprivation* (Oxford University Press, 1981).

by people, but a large fraction of the deaths it has caused, at least in the US, were preventable.[14] As humans take on more and more responsibility in these realms, theological questions around natural disasters may only grow more frequent.

Natural disaster theology has also grown in importance for another reason: the rise of impossibly complex technological systems. The emergence of these systems means that when a human-built system experiences large-scale failure, there may no longer be a single, clear cause. Instead, catastrophes are often the result of a cascade of errors, some of which are unpreventable and many of which appear minor on their own. To pick an example: the 1979 nuclear disaster at Three Mile Island took place because an unusually dirty water filter warranted a cleaning method that caused a water turbine to shut off; because three emergency valves had been closed in violation of a regulation; and because the light on a control panel malfunctioned, leading an operator to release needed coolant from the system. Writing about the disaster, Charles Perrow noted, bleakly, that accidents of these kinds may be so complex that we cannot easily learn from them.[15] If he is correct, then perhaps the modern definition of "natural disaster" includes not just the seemingly-random violence of the natural world, but the expectation of unexpected failures in our artificial worlds, as well.

Here we are, then, in a world that is increasingly dominated by disasters that entangle God and people and the problematic theologies that accompany these entanglements. Much as the Holocaust loomed large in the theologies of the latter half of the previous century, climate change and a catastrophically inept response to a global pandemic are the toxic soil out of which all 21st century theologies must grow. If we do not wish to leave theology to the politicians, it is incumbent upon us to formulate something stronger that is articulated not just reactively in a frantic gasp to give meaning to death, but in a way that allows us to hold both God and human beings to account.

---

[14] Irwin Redlener et al., "'130,000 – 210,000 Avoidable COVID-19 Deaths – and Counting – in the U.S.,'" 2020.

[15] Charles Perrow, *Normal Accidents: Living with High-Risk Technologies* (New York: Basic Books, 1984).

Two Methods of Disentanglement

I do not have complete answers to these problems, but I'd like to outline two promising arguments by which the entanglement of divine and human responsibility can be dissolved, if not disentangled. One of these arguments has backing from the Jewish philosophical tradition. The other does not.

The more traditional argument is that God can evade blame for natural disasters not because of limits on God's power or knowledge but because God's activity in the world is extraordinarily subtle, and it is therefore not possible to point to incident Y and posit that God effected it for reason X. The most important proponent of this idea was Maimonides (d. 1204), whose *Guide of the Perplexed* (III:32) puts forward the notion that God operates via *talaṭṭuf*, an Arabic term which Samuel Ibn Tibbon (d. 1232) translated as *'orma,* and which Shlomo Pines rendered as "wily graciousness."[16] In context, *talaṭṭuf* is used to explain developments in Jewish custom; for example, the Bible's interest in animal sacrifice is explained as an attempt by God to introduce monotheism in terms that a people fresh from Egyptian slavery would understand.

But *talaṭṭuf*'s explanatory powers extend far beyond resolving textual issues, because another way of saying that God is wily and gracious is saying that God is always keenly aware of the needs of the universe and is always acting to keep them in balance through subtle, precisely determined measures. When read this way, God begins to take on the shape of an ecosystem, one which humans reside within but ultimately do not completely understand or dictate. Pantheist readings of *talaṭṭuf* are possible but not necessary. For our purposes, what matters is that imagining divine action as an ecosystem allows us to impute a logic to it without letting human beings off the hook.

The solution of "wily graciousness" has the benefit of being useful in a climate crisis, but it also has an element of hand-waving to it. Like Rabbi Lord Jakobovits, it places a limit on how well we can ever understand

---

[16] Moses Maimonides, *The Guide of the Perplexed*, ed. Shlomo Pines (Chicago: University of Chicago Press, 1963), lxxii. Note that it is Ibn Tibbon's *'orma* that contains the concept of wiliness, something that is not directly suggested by *talaṭṭuf*. See Pines' note on the reason for this translation. On the "divine ruse," see Amos Funkenstein, *Maimonides: Political Theory and Realistic Messianism* (De Gruyter, 1977), ch. 5.

what is going on, not because it is not our place to inquire, but because we would not understand the answer. It is certainly possible to see this as a distinction without a difference. A second solution avoids this problem, but only does so by introducing a new theological postulate.

In describing the growing relevance of natural disaster theology above, I noted that there are an increasing number of areas where events traditionally associated with God can now be plausibly blamed on humans, leading to a problematic overlapping set of responsibilities. But what if we reject the possibility of overlap—that is, what if we say that natural disasters are *either* God's fault *or* they are our fault? In such a bifurcated domain of responsibility, one would see humanity's territory grow while God's territory shrinks. Humanity, in other words, becomes responsible for an ever-growing number of disasters, while God's responsibility diminishes at the same pace. As we take on God's roles, we take on God's responsibilities, as well—but crucially, these responsibilities are identical in character to the ones we have now. The reason for this is best articulated in a passage from the Babylonian Talmud:

> Rabbi Hama, son of Rabbi Hanina, says: Why is it written, "After the Lord your God shall you walk," (Deut. 13:5)? Is it possible for a person to follow the Divine Presence? Hasn't it already been stated, "For the Lord your God is a devouring fire" (Deut. 4:24). Instead, one should follow the attributes of the Holy Blessed One. Just as God clothes the naked, as it is written, "And the Lord God made for Adam and for his wife garments of skin, and clothed them" (Gen. 3:21), so, too, should you clothe the naked. Just as the Holy Blessed One visits the sick, as it is written [concerning Abraham's circumcision], "And the Lord appeared unto him by the terebinths of Mamre" (Gen. 18:1), so, too, should you visit the sick. Just as the Holy Blessed One consoles mourners, as it is written, "And it came to pass after the death of Abraham, that God blessed Isaac his son" (Gen. 25:11), so, too, should you console mourners. Just as the Holy Blessed One buried the dead, as it is written, "And [Moses] was buried in the valley in the land of Moab" (Deut. 34:6), so,

too, should you bury the dead.[17]

God, like humanity, is engaged in the daily task of caring for others; to take on divine responsibility, then, does not involve a change in the nature of our tasks, but only in the expectation for how we carry them out. If most of the harm that occurs during a natural disaster is caused by humans, there is no theological need to shoehorn God into the blame equation.

In conclusion, let us step back for a moment to consider what this solution does for us. In understanding ourselves as the causes of erstwhile divine events, we can avoid fraught theologies and bad policies, and we can even charge human beings with new and greater moral responsibilities. But, to return to the storm gods of the ancients, we ought to remember that this is not a theological footnote, but an update to a belief that stems from the core desire to find meaning in the events that literally shape the world around us.

Both the problems and solutions raised here suggest that this role can no longer be maintained. But theology, ultimately, is pneumatic; if God can no longer be in the hurricane, other homes are surely available. While this might direct God outward, to effects still beyond our control, like asteroid impacts, it is, perhaps, the fate of natural disaster theology to push God much closer to us, to circumstances that are not widely shared, that affect no one but ourselves. There may still be worlds shaken by God. Perhaps they are just not the ones we had in mind.

---

[17] b. Sotah 14a.

Between Immanence and Transcendence:
Jewish Ideas of God and Suffering

Rachel Sabath Beit-Halachmi

Uncertainty, crises, tragedy, and sustained suffering are hardly new experiences in Jewish life. In every period of Jewish history, Jews have faced significant calamities of one kind or another, so it is no surprise that Jewish canonical texts and prayers reflect many responses to such experiences. Some prayers, like those many Jews recite daily or weekly celebrating the Exodus from ancient Egypt, praise God and God's divine might for redeeming the Jewish people from slavery. Other prayers, like those said on Hanukkah or Purim, are triumphant—recalling attempts in different historic periods to annihilate the Jewish people and their miraculous survival nonetheless. Biblical texts, like those in Psalms or the Book of Lamentations, call upon God to take notice of individual or collective suffering and plead for healing, strength, and support.

Just as there are infinite ways in which human beings respond to the experience of love, so too are there infinite responses to the experience of suffering. Jewish responses vary greatly in their attitude toward suffering, their theological understanding of the meaning or purpose of suffering, and their understanding of God and God's power (or lack thereof). The current pandemic is no different. It has already generated its own diversity of Jewish responses. This essay will consider the relevance of ancient and modern theological responses to prior crises to the experience of suffering and plague in our time, and will outline several categories of Jewish responses that are already emerging.

1. Ancient, Medieval, Modern, and Postmodern Responses to Suffering: Why Does God Let Us Suffer? The Eternal Human Question

The range of Jewish responses to suffering is immense: the repeated calls of the enslaved Israelites to God to notice their suffering in ancient

Egypt;[1] the responses to the destruction of the first and second Temples in the Book of Lamentations; the trials of centuries of exile recorded in *piyyut* (liturgical poetry) and *tekhines*;[2] the more recent responses to the Shoah (Holocaust).[3] Whether the response is religious or secular—in Hebrew or another language—these texts demonstrate the ongoing and profound human need to put into words the specific yet universal pain and experience of rupture.

Some responses to crises express anger. In several Psalms, for example, the author asks, "*Ad matai?!* [How long will this suffering continue?]" (Ps. 74:1); or, "How long, God, will you hide Your face from us?" (Ps. 13:1). As the Christian Bible scholar Walter Brueggemann teaches, to have an authentic relationship with God, we must present our real selves, "not compliant false selves that conceal pain and anger behind a pleasant mask."[4] The Book of Psalms is the record of a truthful relationship between embodied, fragile humans who inhabit an unpredictable world and a God who is intermittently present for and sometimes terrifyingly absent from its inhabitants (Ps. 13:1, for example). In addition to the Psalms, expressions of yearning for, rage at, and even denial of God's existence can be found throughout the Bible, the Book of Lamentations—and most dramatically, in the Book of Job.

Commentators throughout the ages offer a wide spectrum of responses to ancient narratives of tragedy, whether or not redemption ensued. Some glorify God and God's power, while others describe God as hidden. Some believe that in our suffering God is exceedingly close to us but powerless to intervene; others see the loss of innocent lives as proof of God's absence—maybe even God's death. Indeed, contradicting interpretations of God's power or presence or existence can be found even on the same page of text. This multivocality—especially in a time of crisis—is part of the pluralism of the Jewish tradition. While one text might sing out and praise

---

[1] Exod. 2:23-24

[2] Tekhines (Yiddish for tekhinot or supplications) are private devotional prayers in Yiddish written by women and men and recited primarily by women. They were first authored beginning in 1600, became popular between 1700-1900, and continue to be written, collected, and recited today.

[3] See, for example, Michael L. Morgan's *Beyond Auschwitz: Post Holocaust Jewish Thought in America*. (Oxford: Oxford University Press, 2001).

[4] Walter Brueggemann, "The Costly Loss of Lament," *JSOT* 36 (1986): 49-56.

God for the redemption from Egypt, another text reprimands the angels for singing while the Sea of Reeds closes around the Egyptian pursuers. According to the Sages, God scolded them, saying, "How dare you sing for joy when My creatures are dying?!" (b. Megillah 10b; b. Sanhedrin 39b). On a ritual level, when we celebrate a wedding and the creation of a Jewish home, we break a glass to remember the destruction of God's Home, the Temple in Jerusalem (Tosafot on b. Berachot 31a). Jewish thought and practice insist on holding dialectical approaches together.

2. The Transcendent or the Immanent God? Dialectical Views of God in the Face of Tragedy

Theological Questions in a Time of Crises

The experience of unjust suffering, especially when children and other clearly innocent people suffer, has led to profound theological questions from biblical times to the present. Is God great, doing wonders, omnipotent in every aspect of human history? Are the tragedies we experience part of a grand plan that only God understands? Has God hidden God's face (hester panim) now, as God has done before? Can we get to the other side of that? Was God once a powerful actor in human history, but now no longer able to influence the disasters of the natural world, much less stop the atrocities of human beings? Or is God not so far away from the suffering human being, but rather immanent—with us in our suffering? Does God even hear our cries? Can God change our circumstances? Finally, we ask again in our suffering, why does God allow such horrific things to happen to good people? If God loves us, why can't God save us? Is it because of something we did? Is our suffering meant to teach us something about how we need to change in the future?

Do We Suffer Because God is Punishing Us? Or Because God Loves Us?

The Sages of the Talmud discuss these questions at great length in several different passages. One view is that suffering is a direct divine response to human transgression. Sin yields punishment. Distraction from Torah study yields retribution. However, should one not be able to identify wrongdoing, there is yet another possible explanation for pain: *yissurin shel ahavah*—afflictions of love. God only brings such afflictions to those God loves, perhaps to purify or to inspire repentance. The Talmud states:

> Rava, and some say Rav Hisda, said: If a person sees that suffering has befallen him, he should examine his actions, as it is stated: "We will search and examine our ways, and return to God" (Lam. 3:40). If he examined his ways and found no transgression for which that suffering is appropriate, he may attribute his suffering to dereliction in the study of Torah, as it is stated: "Happy is the man whom You punish, Lord, and teach out of Your law" (Ps. 94:12). And if he did attribute his suffering to dereliction in the study of Torah, and did not find anything, he may be confident that these are afflictions of love, as it is stated: "For whom the Lord loves, He rebukes" (Prov. 3:12). (b. Berakhot 5a)

In reading such passages, one might rightly ask whether suffering is a sign of human sin or a sign of God's love. Could one really know? In what way could suffering be a sign of God's love? Are those afflicted in this pandemic more loved by God than those who are not? In most traditional commentaries, the response to these questions is that whether or not a plague or another type of suffering is a sign of God's love, one must continue to be vigilant in observance and not question God's ways.

One contemporary instantiation of this perplexing mode of thinking can be found in the words of a British Modern Orthodox rabbi who explains that the suffering of our present pandemic is both "the cost of biological diversity" which is "disease and infection" *and* a sign of God being "a loving and enabling teacher."

> We only rebuke the ones we love, because they matter to us the most. And we only truly accept rebuke from those that love us, because we know that they have our best interests at heart. The way I see it, God created this world with infinite diversity

and complexity. A garden of opportunity for us all. But the cost of biological diversity is disease and infection. God built this into nature. The only question is how you respond to it, as Rabbi Hanina said, "All is in the hands of Heaven, except for the reverence of Heaven" (b. Berakhot 33b). We always have a choice how to respond to what happens to us…I see God as a loving and enabling teacher rather than an authoritarian school master. This terrible virus is not a punishment. It is what it is.[5]

"It is what it is" is a tempting conclusion for a theodicy that might implicate God or cause protest against God. At times when God's presence and goodness are most needed, very few Jewish thinkers want to open the door for profound theological protest against God, whether because of God's hiddenness, God's powerlessness, or—God forbid!—God's non-existence. From the perspective of those who uphold a transcendent God who cannot stop specific suffering because the natural world God created proceeds as it must (an idea known in rabbinic literature as *"olam k'minhago noheg"* (b. Avodah Zarah 54b)), God always remains all-powerful, utterly righteous, and beyond reproach. Many embrace this theology because it makes room for a God who allows righteous people to suffer—either because God knows reasons we cannot fathom, or because in God's creation of the world, there is a natural order which is set—even if it means that suffering of the innocent ensues. In response, we human beings should not hold God responsible, question God, be angry at God, or lose faith in God.

In ancient and modern Jewish theology, however, there is simultaneously a very different possible understanding of God: a view that God is not far away, transcendent and beyond reach, but rather that God is immanent—very near to us and even with us in our suffering. If the ancient Israelites are suffering and weeping, God is weeping with them. If the Jews are crying out to God because they are enslaved, exiled or oppressed, God hears their cry and suffers with them. If the Jews are being dragged out of the Land of Israel in the first century, or toward the crematoria of

---

[5] Raphael Zarum, "If Everything Comes from God What Does that Say about the Coronavirus?" The Jewish Chronicle, Sept. 24, 2020.

Auschwitz in the twentieth century, God, too, is in chains and experiences that exile together with the Jewish people.

3. Reinterpreting Talmudic Text in Light of the Pandemic

Rabbinic literature—all of Jewish literature, for that matter—is not lacking for crisis narratives. In most cases, toward the end of the narrative, the reader learns how God (or a representative angel, a voice from heaven, or a prophet of God) views such a response. Many of these narratives portray a transcendent God, while others show a more immanent God. Abraham Joshua Heschel (1907-1972), the great modern theologian, in his three-volume *tour de force* entitled *Torah MinHashamayim b'Aspaklariyah shel HaDorot* (*Heavenly Torah: As Refracted through the Generations*) interprets hundreds of texts to elucidate the theology of the Sages. In Heschel's view, the plurality of ancient Jewish theological approaches to God, especially given the sheer volume of rabbinic voices arguing alternately for the transcendent or the immanent, is indicative of the deep roots of pluralism in Jewish thought—and therefore the pluralism that should be inherent in Jewish life.[6]

Of the many possible texts one could bring from the Talmud, there is a text that is particularly relevant for this time of pandemic and quarantine.[7] In Tractate Shabbat there are many narratives that tell of the dramatic and horrific challenges that the Sages of the first century in the Land of Israel faced during and after the siege of Jerusalem and the destruction of the Second Temple (c. 70 CE) by the Romans. A strange but very relevant passage tells a long story about Rabbi Shimon Bar Yohai and his son, R. Eleazar, who hide in a cave for twelve years in order to be able to continue to study Torah. The Roman authorities forbade Torah study on pain of death by torture (as was the case with Rabbi Akiva). In the cave,

---

[6] Abraham Joshua Heschel, *Torah MinHashamayim b'Aspaklariyah shel HaDorot* (New York: Soncino Press, 1962). *Heavenly Torah: As Refracted through the Generations*, ed. & trans. Gordon Tucker (London: Continuum, 2004).

[7] Other Talmudic narratives relevant to the current pandemic include the story in Tr. Gittin 56b, in which Yohanan ben Zakkai barely escapes from a besieged Jerusalem to create a new rabbinic academy in Yavneh. It is a story of dispute and risk-taking for the sake of building something new, rather than allowing Judaism to fade away in the wake of the destruction of Jerusalem by the Romans.

miracles happened:

> A miracle occurred and a carob-tree and a water well were created for them.

> They would strip their garments and sit up to their necks in sand. The whole day they studied; when it was time for prayers they robed, covered themselves, prayed, and then put off their garments again, so that they should not wear out. Thus they dwelt twelve years in the cave. (b. Shabbat 33b)

The two are forced back into the world by none other than Elijah the prophet—who had to come get them because they were so removed from society that they did not even know that the Roman decree had been lifted. But their long quarantine had changed them; being in the world was intolerable to them.

> Whatever they cast their eyes upon was immediately burnt up. Thereupon a Heavenly Voice came forth and cried out, "Have you emerged to destroy My world?! Return to your cave!" So they returned and dwelt there twelve months, as punishment. "I did not invite you out of the cave in order to destroy my world! Go back in; return to your cave," [said God]…" (b. Shabbat 33b)

The two spend eleven more months in the cave and ultimately emerge more able to function in the world. But the critique is clear: abandoning the world entirely in order to study Torah while denying the human body and the needs of society is not at all what God wants.

Ultimately, withdrawing from society totally is not only ineffective; it is also destructive. Separating oneself from the community—another prohibition in rabbinic literature (Ethics of the Ancestors 2:4)—so completely for so long, even for the sake of Torah study, leads to one being cut off from the community of the people of Israel and unable to participate in its daily life. Self-isolation and asceticism face criticism in many contexts of Jewish textual tradition, but here it is an internal criticism within the narrative itself. Only if that separation or hiding is for the sake of *pikuach nefesh* (saving a life) is it permissible, and only for the shortest possible amount of time.

This anti-isolationist stance raises tensions for us today. For much of this pandemic, hiding in the cave of one's home has been the only rational way to weather the dangerous storm outside. And yet foundational aspects of Jewish communal life have pulled on us to gather. In some parts of the Jewish community, the idea of a transcendent and all-powerful God has translated into gathering together for communal prayer, even in the face of medical advice and government decrees to stay home. For this population, God will ultimately determine "who shall live and who shall die." The job of human beings is to search their deeds to understand why they are being punished; to understand their suffering as a sign of God's love. For others, both in the Bible and in the modern Jewish experience, laying blame at the feet of someone else is paramount—be it foreigners, people of another faith, or people of another Jewish denomination. Finally, some leaders in the Jewish community, privileging physical safety, encouraged "cave dwelling" while cultivating communal ties through technological means.

Sadly, the social distance and isolation have been ongoing and the consequences are likely building, though it is much too soon to begin to analyze the long-term impact on different parts of the community and on human life and faith in general. Judaism, whether in a context of glory or in suffering, is a system that creates islands of the sacred regardless of what is happening in the outside world. At the same time, modern Jewish thinkers emphasize that, at its core, there is no affirmation or encouragement in Judaism to abandon society. On the contrary, we are charged to engage and remedy it.

4. Where is God in the Current Pandemic?

In the current pandemic, Jewish thinkers, as well as those of other traditions, have suggested similar ideas: Either the pandemic has come to punish us for our sins, or to purify us, or as a sign of God's great love for the Jewish People, the suffering remnant. Pope Francis, among others, argued that Covid-19 is nature's response to humans ignoring the current climate crisis.[8] Most non-Orthodox rabbis who have been asked if Covid-19 is a punishment from God for our sins respond that it clearly is not. Liberal Jews generally do not believe in reward and punishment as such, and do not believe that a suffering person is helped in any way by being blamed for or being accused of having caused their own suffering. If one thinks that God is directly involved in such a pandemic, it is understandable that one might ask, "What kind of God would unleash such a horrific disease that attacks our very breath?" Rather most modern Jews understand that the virus and its impact are a product of biological processes. In other words, "it's biology, not theology." God may be all-powerful as the creator of the universe, but God created a world that functions according to natural laws, *"olam k'minhago noheg."* While prayers and Jewish teachings might offer support or even hope, "right now we need doctors and vaccines, not rabbis and sermons."[9]

At the same time, others—including the present author—believe that while the cruel virus and its disease may be a product of the natural world, we must still embrace what it can teach us. It teaches us not only about the precarious nature of the climate and the interaction between the human and animal worlds, but also about our strengths and weaknesses as a human society. The pandemic shines a bright light to show where our human social fabric is strong and where it is threadbare. Among other stark realizations we in the United States, in particular, have become painfully aware of the failures of our health system; of economic injustice and systemic racism; and of how the impact of each of these social ills is compounded by the impact of a pandemic. On a global scale we have become profoundly aware of stark economic and racial inequalities and of widespread starvation and death that could be prevented.

In sermons during the High Holy Days of 2020, as it became clear that the pandemic was killing hundreds of thousands of people in the U.S. and many more around the world, and that the suffering would continue for an indefinite amount of time, North American liberal rabbis focused on the texts and Jewish theology that would affirm God's presence and God's

---

[8] CNN News, "Pope says coronavirus pandemic could be nature's response to climate crisis," April 9, 2020. https://www.cnn.com/2020/04/08/europe/pope-francis-coronavirus-nature-response-intl/index.html.

[9] Zarum, "If Everything Comes from God…" (See note 5).

caring immanence. More than one rabbi taught the following midrash:

> "There once was a man on a journey who came across a beautiful palace, but the palace was on fire. He looked around, trying to find help to put out the blaze. He wondered, surely there must someone who owns this palace, someone who cares for it. This, the rabbis teach in the midrash (Genesis Rabbah 39:1), was our ancestor Abraham. And the palace on fire, the *birah doleket*, was the world itself.
>
> Seeing the world on fire, the world consumed by chaos and corruption, Abraham looked around for someone to put out the flames. He asked, surely there must be someone in charge of this burning world. Surely there must be someone who cares for it. And that's when he heard God's voice calling to him: I am the caretaker of this palace, 'I am the Sovereign of the universe. *Lech Lecha*, go forth from your land, you will start a great nation and I will be your God.' (Gen. 12:1)[10]

This midrash presents a possible third mode of theological struggle with God when the world is on fire. While God cannot stop the fire, God has chosen Abraham—and by extension, the Jewish people—to put out the fire. Yes, God is the great Creator of the Universe, but God has created a world which will follow its natural course, *olam k'minhago noheg*. When we human beings act ethically, in partnership with God, we can limit the impact of crises and decrease human suffering.

5. The Postmodern Turn: New Ways to Understand God in a Time of Crises

In the twentieth century, new articulations of Jewish theology emerged in prose and poetry, in rituals and liturgies. The periods of greatest creativity have occurred during times of widespread anguish during and

---

[10] Rachel Timoner, "Who By Fire," Rosh Hashanah Sermon, Sept. 2020. Text and video available at: https://www.sefaria.org/sheets/265140?lang=bi. For a variety of other sermons that reflect similar concerns during the High Holy Days 2020: https://www.myjewishlearning.com/category/celebrate/rosh-hashanah/rosh-hashanah-yom-kippur-coronavirus/.

especially following the persecution and murder of more than six million Jews during the Holocaust; in the midst of losses weathered by Israelis during its many wars of survival and conflicts; and during and following ongoing antisemitic clashes in many parts of the world. The Holocaust, for example, revived eternal questions about God and suffering. For some, like the main character in Elie Wiesel's well-known volume *Night,* God is dead, hanging in the gallows of Auschwitz.[11] Though not a survivor himself, the radical theologian Richard Rubenstein (b. 1924) declared the Holocaust the beginning of the death of God. In Rubenstein's first book, *After Auschwitz: Radical Theology and Contemporary Judaism* (1966), published just a few years after Wiesel's *Night* first appeared in English, Rubenstein explored radical ideas in Jewish theology. He argued that the experience of the Holocaust shattered the traditional Jewish concept of God, especially as the God of the covenant with Abraham, in which the God of Israel is the God of history. Rubenstein argued that Jews could no longer advocate the notion of an omnipotent God at work in history or espouse the election of Israel as the chosen people. In the wake of the Holocaust, he believed that Jews have lost hope and that there is no ultimate meaning to life. "I am compelled to say that we live in the time of the 'death of God.' This is more a statement about man and his culture than about God. The death of God is a cultural fact."[12]

Many traditional Jewish theologians, however, returned to more familiar tropes of Jewish theology in response to the Holocaust. Eliezer Berkovits (1908-1992), in a book called *Faith After the Holocaust,* argues in the introduction that one must not judge the theology of anyone who suffers.[13] A person cannot judge a survivor, just as the Bible teaches that one cannot judge Job, in all of his suffering and all of his responses—for we are not Job. Rather, suggests Berkovits, we are Job's cousin. From this familial stance, Berkovits suggests a very close and caring relationship to Job—the one who actually suffers—yet a clear distinction between that person and the rest of us, the ones who gaze upon that person as they suffer or who live in another time and place. One cannot possibly know

---

[11] Elie Wiesel, Night (New York: Hill & Wang, 1960).

[12] Richard Rubenstein, *After Auschwitz* (Indianapolis, IN: Bobbs-Merrill Publishers, 1966), 18.

[13] Eliezer Berkovits, *Faith After the Holocaust* (New York: KTAV Publishing House, 1973).

what questions we would ask of God or what blasphemy we would speak of God if we were in that particular horrific situation, God forbid. In other words, explains Berkovits, one cannot judge the theology of those Jews who marched to the gas chambers having lost their faith or, alternately, those who declared their faith—"I believe," *Ani Ma'amin*[14]—in the same situation. There are survivors who speak of how their faith in a transcendent, omnipotent God grew even stronger, as Job's did. And others, like the victims and survivors Wiesel speaks of and writes about, who, in their horrific suffering, lost their faith in God. All responses are legitimate in the ever-widening field of Jewish theology.

In contrast, Eugene B. Borowitz (1924-2016) argued that what died in the Holocaust was not God, but rather the "false Messiah of modernity." In Borowitz's postmodern Jewish thought, God was not a casualty of the Nazis; faith in human beings was. It was the worship of the human mind and of "human progress" that to a large extent enabled and perpetuated the annihilation of six million Jews and millions of other human beings, and so it was this faith that was destroyed in the Shoah.[15] Taking a very different but related stance on the theological implications of genocide, Irving (Yitz) Greenberg argued that after the Shoah, the covenant between God and the Jewish people can only be a "voluntary covenant."[16]

David Blumenthal (b. 1938) published a volume of "radical" theology entitled *Facing the Abusing God: A Theology of Protest*. Blumenthal argues that having faith in a post-Holocaust world means "admitting that while God is often loving and kind, fair and merciful, God is also capable of acts so unjust they can only be described as abusive." Blumenthal grounds his argument in biblical texts, and in the experience of Holocaust survivors and survivors of child abuse. Blumenthal brings together the challenge of facing a God who works "wondrously through us" and who has worked "aw(e)fully against us.[17] This is another framing of the spectrum of im-

---

[14] Maimonides, Thirteen Principles of Jewish Faith, Chapter 9, 156-163.

[15] Eugene B. Borowitz, *Renewing the Covenant: A Theology for the Postmodern Jew* (Philadelphia: Jewish Publication Society, 1991), 18-19; 79; 232.

[16] Irving Greenberg, "Voluntary Covenant," in Perspectives (New York: CLAL: The National Jewish Center for Learning and Leadership, 1987). The original version can be found here: https://rabbiirvinggreenberg.com/wp-content/uploads/2013/02/2Perspectives-Voluntary-Covenant-1987-CLAL-2-of-3.pdf

[17] David Blumenthal, *Facing the Abusing God: A Theology of Protest* (Louisville, KY: Westminster/John Knox Press, 1993), 267.

manent and transcendent ideas about God in the context of the suffering of the innocent.

In her path-breaking work *Engendering Judaism: An Inclusive Theology and Ethics,* Rachel Adler (b. 1943) offers new ways of understanding God's immanent presence in prayer, in contemporary ethical decision making, in the experiences of suffering and loneliness, and the joy of entering into a covenant of love. The engendered Judaism she seeks is one that must achieve a number of goals through multiple methodologies and disciplines simultaneously: "We will have to make the theological project as complicated as the world from which we launch it. This requires not *a* method but an entire repertory of methods for thinking, for reading, for describing, and for imagining how diversely situated and gendered people have lived, do live and could live Jewish lives."[18] Adler is also well known for creating a new non-*ketubah* (traditional Jewish legal document) for Jewish weddings. She wrote the text to describe the covenant of a truly egalitarian partnership and she called this new marriage covenant a *Brit Ahuvim,* a Covenant of Lovers. Her work provides the groundwork for rethinking and reimagining how Jewish texts can speak to a new reality, whether it be one of egalitarianism or a new era of lament, such as an unprecedented global pandemic.

This provides the context in which to approach a later paper Adler wrote specifically about the textual resources for a theology of suffering entitled "'For These I Weep:' A Theology of Lament." In it, Adler argues, "Because God is a God of justice and not a cosmic bully, God can be confronted by God's covenant partner...Rather than presenting a compliant false self and rendering the relationship manipulative and insincere, the lamenter confronts God with the immediacy of suffering in a way that renders retribution unjustifiable."[19] Adler points to well-known Christian Bible scholar Walter Brueggemann's concept of lament. Brueggemann understands lament as a way of communicating with God that shifts the calculus between the human being and God.[20] The one who expresses

---

[18] Rachel Adler, *Engendering Judaism: An Inclusive Theology and Ethics* (Philadelphia: Jewish Publication Society, 1998; Boston: Beacon Press, 1999), xxiii.

[19] Adler, "'For These I Weep:' A Theology of Lament," The Chronicle, March 2006.

[20] Walter Brueggemann, "The Costly Loss of Lament," JSOT 36 (1986) 49-56. See also: Brueggemann, "A Shape for Old Testament Theology, II: Embrace of Pain," The Catholic Biblical Quarterly 47, no. 3 (1985): 395-415. Accessed March 16, 2021. http://www.jstor.

their suffering through this kind of crying out shifts the distribution of power between the two parties so that the human being, the petitionary party, is taken seriously. As Adler explains: "The God rooted in the Book of Lamentations emphasizes and authorizes human beings—especially suffering human beings—to bring anger and frustration and lament into their prayer and theology."[21] Lament in a liturgical context, as recorded in these and many other sacred texts, becomes the foundation on which modern thinkers as well as contemporary theologians and the creative liturgists of our time create new responses.

6. Some Early Jewish Theological Responses to Covid-19

It is much too soon to comprehend the long-term spiritual impact of this pandemic while we are still in the midst of it. At the same time, we have already witnessed extensive responses to this new reality in every sphere of Jewish life. Many follow the contours of what we outlined above: a range of transcendent and immanent ideas about God and suffering. While the challenges of the current pandemic continue, we also continue to gain a broader and deeper understanding of the shifting and deepening role of religion in the lives of human beings who are suffering and mourning in our time.

Some of the new thinking has emerged out of necessity because of new *halakhic* (legal) considerations, both in the Orthodox and non-Orthodox segments of the Jewish community. Some new halakhic questions included whether a *minyan* (a prayer quorum of ten adult Jews) can be counted while each person is in a separate location, seen and heard only through technology and a screen. What about the mourner's *Kaddish*? What about for a funeral? What if it is declared unsafe to gather even at a distance? Even with masks? What about on Shabbat? Can one leave the Zoom running and untouched for those who don't use technology during the Sabbath? Different segments of the Jewish community answered

---

org/stable/43716986.

[21] Adler, "'For These I Weep:' A Theology of Lament," The Chronicle, March 2006; and Adler, "Two Psalms for Hard Times You Won't Find in Your Prayerbook," Scriptions: Jewish Thought and Response to Covid-19; https://scriptions.huc.edu/scriptions/two-psalms-for-hard-times-you-wont-find-in-your-prayerbook. October 2020.

these questions differently, and at times even changed their responses and widened the possibilities of Jewish collective prayer and ritual.

In addition, previously practiced rituals were reinvented or repurposed. Calls went out for a worldwide Jewish community recitation of Psalms at precisely the same time. "Though I walk through the valley of death I shall fear I fear nothing because God is with me…." (Ps. 23) was uttered by thousands of Jews simultaneously, all able to see their far-flung prayer partners on Zoom. In other moments in the early months of the coronavirus, there was also a call for a worldwide fast day to plead with God, a practice originally established in rabbinic literature as a communal response in a time of famine or drought. In an open letter, Ashkenazi Chief Rabbi David Lau called for a fast day of at least half a day on March 25, 2020 in response to the coronavirus epidemic. "The Jewish people are suffering, as is the entire world. At this time, we must engage in soul searching," he wrote. In early April 2020, before Passover, chief rabbis worldwide launched #KeepingItTogether Shabbat. It was a campaign to make this Shabbat before Passover, known as Shabbat HaGadol, "a Shabbat of kindness, a Shabbat of prayer and a Shabbat of connection to the Divine."[22] In addition to these Jewish communal responses, there were interfaith gatherings to recite Psalm 23 and Psalm 121, including a gathering in Jerusalem on April 15, 2020.[23]

Between March 2020 and ongoing to the publication of this essay, countless additional *kavanot* have been written in response to the pandemic. These are individual and collective prayers to be read when reading Torah in the absence of a Torah scroll; when praying at home alone; when praying on Zoom or other online platforms. Additional prayers for the sick have continued to appear, as well as prayers for the caregivers.[24] An enormous collection of rituals, classes, lectures, prayers, and music events have been available online. This time of pandemic has witnessed the massive growth of new modes of learning across time and space. The new platform of JewishLIVE.org, for example, has seen ongoing growth

---

[22] See overview of such events in Jewish Times, https://www.jewishtimes.com/105052/jta-roundup-latest-coronavirus-news-from-jewish-communities-around-the-world/news/.

[23] See, for example, Marcy Oster, "Religious Leaders in Jerusalem Recite Joint Prayer Composed for Coronavirus," https://www.timesofisrael.com/religious-leaders-in-jerusalem-recite-joint-prayer-composed-for-coronavirus/.

[24] See, for example: https://www.ritualwell.org/ritual/caregivers-prayer.

in the type and sheer volume of people gathering online for myriad different kinds of Jewish learning in every time zone, not limited by geography. Most of these ritual, liturgical, and educational efforts call upon an immanent God to be with those who are suffering, to give strength to the professionals and families caretaking, and to bring comfort to the unfathomable number of people mourning. They perform and embody the dictum of Rabbi Abraham Isaac Kook (1865-1935): "The old shall be made new and the new shall be made holy."[25]

Considering the past year of plague and pandemic, we might understand this creativity and ritual adjustment as having occurred in stages. As of the writing of this essay, one can already identify several major types of Jewish ritual and theological response, aligned loosely with the developing timeline of the pandemic, now more than a full year into killing millions of people around the world. In North America, the early phase might be named "A Radical Pause and a Passover Seder on Zoom." In March-April of 2020 there was a dramatic break in Jewish life exemplified by the experience of gathering on Zoom for Seder, in stark contrast to the ingathering that usually marks the Passover holiday. But the spring of adaptations was followed by what one might call a "Summer of Death and Hope." The death tolls were mounting exponentially; at the same time, there were glimmers of hope in the positive results of various vaccine trials.[26] Having adapted to online prayer and ritual, some felt strengthened anew by their faith and by the now broader experience of community made possible by technology. It had already become common that those who attended online prayer services and celebrations and participated in shiva gatherings could do so across time zones and geographic separation. The fall of 2020 was characterized by a frenzy of discontented searches to create new ways to mark the High Holy Days in isolation or lockdown. This was the beginning of what many called the "New Normal." This new reality created by the pandemic generated even more creativity, including new liturgy and new modes of celebrating. But whatever new normalcy may have been begrudgingly accepted in the short term, it was followed

---

[25] Binyamin Ish Shalom, *Rav Avraham Itzhak HaCohen Kook: Between Rationalism and Mysticism* (Albany: State University of New York Press, 1993), 12.

[26] Several news sources began reporting hopeful signs of effective vaccines in April 2020. See, for example: https://www.theguardian.com/world/2020/apr/06/when-will-coronavirus-vaccine-be-ready.

by what can only be called a "Winter of Worldwide Catastrophe," as the cases and fatalities continued to grow. With the introduction of a vaccine in early 2021, more *kavanot* and prayers for receiving and administering the vaccine are now emerging. One example of this type of creative theological response to the new experience of receiving a vaccine can be found in the description and the prayer of Miriam Stewart, MD, posted on RitualWell.org where one can also find numerous other rituals and liturgical pieces created for this ongoing time of pandemic.

> As I was waiting in line for the Covid-19 vaccine I was quite nervous but also filled with gratitude for human ingenuity and the collective will to survive and protect each other. I was reflecting on the Hebrew word for vaccine—*hisun*—which shares a root with the word *yehesayun*—meaning protection or refuge —from one of my favorite phrases of Psalm 36:8: "In the shadow of Your wings humankind finds protection" (or shelter or refuge—whichever word resonates most for you).
>
> As the needle entered my skin—with all the hope and uncertainty it represents—this blessing came to me: *Im hisun zeh b'tzel kenafekha yehesayun*: "With this vaccine, may we be protected in the shadow of Your wings." When I go to get my second dose, I'm going to wear my *tallit* (prayer shawl) and say this blessing again, because receiving this vaccine feels like a gift from the universe, an act of faith, and a sacred obligation—a *mitzvah* (commandment)—all at once.[27]

In this newly created ritual, based on ancient words and cloaked in ritual garb, Dr. Stewart has exemplified the idea of the immanent God, the one who is not only nearby protecting us under God's wings, but is as near to us as the fluid of the vaccine entering our arm.

Each crisis shows a community who and what it really is. Crises push us to develop new creative capacities and theological expressions. They reveal

---

[27] Miriam Steward, MD., "In the Shadow of Your Wings: Blessing on Receiving COVID-19 Vaccine." https://www.ritualwell.org/ritual/shadow-your-wings-blessing-receiving-covid-19-vaccine.

the strengths and the weaknesses of particular societies, highlighting the extent to which all have access to basic necessities, care, and healing. The prayers and rituals a person or community recites embody their attempts to make spiritual sense of the world into which they are thrown. These responses are apparent at every point along the transcendent-immanent spectrum, in every context. In this current pandemic crisis in particular, it seems that these theological perspectives are, like so much else, not really binary at all. Because of the pandemic we can see more clearly who we are as a human society, and what each of our sub-communities, including different sub-communities of the Jewish community, values most. Crisis forces human beings to clarify who we are, how we understand God, and who we want to be—if we survive—and often generates more attempts to speak out toward and with that God. In order for new prayers and rituals to be authentic, these new expressions of theology will, as Adler insists, be "as complicated as the world from which we launch it."[28]

Crisis, our Eternal Teacher—during which one might understand God to be loving or punishing, warm and comforting, or distant and cruel—demands that the community rise to care for each other. Crisis can also spur the growth of the human soul. Each person of faith—including those who wrestle with God, shout laments to God, protest against God, abandon their faith, or embrace God's love in some way—can find in crisis the opportunity to grow, to engage in deep self-examination, and ultimately enlarge one's spiritual connection to God and to other human beings. Remarkably, the search for God's strength, power, presence, embrace, forgiveness, empathy, and love is a common factor throughout history—and the current pandemic is no exception. As Rabbi Simon, an ancient sage said: "There isn't a single blade of grass that doesn't have a force emanating from heaven to push it and say to it, 'Grow!'"[29]

---

[28] Adler, *Engendering Judaism*, xxiii.
[29] Genesis Rabbah 10:6

The Biblical Plagues and Our Plague:
An Anthropocentric "Theology"

Chaim Seidler-Feller

"Surely there is no fear of God (*yirat Elohim*) in this place."
—Genesis 20:11

The onset of the coronavirus brought with it a slew of perverse efforts to identify the "sinful" behaviors that had occasioned God's wrathful punishment in the form of the global pandemic that had assailed us. In this essay I propose to offer an alternative understanding of "punishment" according to which, rather than being a disciplinary response of the Divine to our transgressions, punishment is actually a fate that befalls us as a direct consequence of our own human conduct. The Egyptian plague narrative will serve as the background for my effort to challenge the classic theological model of reward and punishment, and I will draw on an innovative reading of both biblical sources and Maimonidean philosophy to make my case. Finally, I will outline the corrective program involving a reorientation of our values and a refocusing of our priorities that will be grounded in the fundamental ethical principles of the Jewish tradition.

What God Hath Wrought!

The advent of the pandemic precipitated a range of explanations for a lethal outbreak that was seemingly uncontrollable and had all the markings of an ancient plague. The religious traditionalists could not restrain their predisposition to portray the natural event as divine reproach for one sin or another. These masters of the "ways of heaven" proposed a diverse array of violations that indict humanity which, perversely, justify some form of godly punishment. However, the overwhelming majority of explications bear no direct relationship to the virus itself and can in no rational way be causally linked to the pandemic. They include, among others, a lack of modesty by women (of course), slanderous gossip, and a world sinking ever lower in its commitment to virtue—which necessitated a divine time out. Among the ingenious connections to the virus that have been suggested are the following: since both "corona epidemic" (מגיפת קורונה) and "lack of modesty" (חוסר צניעות) share a numerical value of 900, therefore the virus constitutes a punishment for flagrant breaches of modesty and, since the number of letters in the Ten Commandments equals 620 which is the numerical equivalent of *keter* (crown/*corona*), hence the pandemic could be "a divine message reminding us that we have been given our lives to invest them with meaning and virtue as defined by God's 10 Commandments." This last theodicy was proposed by none other than the Modern Orthodox Rabbi Benjamin Blech! Still other intimates of the Divine Will aver that "*Hashem* is clearly preparing us for *mashiach*, by causing us to observe 14-day periods of quarantine so that we get accustomed to the concept of purity and impurity in anticipation of the rebuilding of the Temple."

Not to be outdone, and occupying a singular position of religious corruption, *Shas* political activists in Israel have taken to offering charms and other forms of "divine protection" against the virus as a campaign gimmick. In a similar vein, early May saw the *Kupat Ha'ir* charitable organization based in Bnei Brak promising donors that if they send in NIS 3000 ($850) they will receive an amulet in addition to an assurance by the foremost Lithuanian Haredi sage Rabbi Chaim Kanievsky that they "will not get sick and that there will not be anyone sick in their home."[1]

The glaring inability to deal with the seeming randomness of and uncertainty engendered by the virus occasioned this rush to explain the true divine justice represented by the calamity that has befallen humanity. Ironically, these religionists who tell themselves and others that they are defending and justifying God and the religious order are actually expressing an inordinate amount of arrogance assuming, as they are, the right and the ability to reveal God's intentions and to pacify their adherents by propounding a quasi-deterministic framework that allays their fears and establishes that Someone is in charge. There is indeed cause and effect, they argue: God is the cause who is bringing about a "legitimate" punishment which can be avoided by following *our* directives. The in-

---

[1] All quotations regarding Orthodox responses to the virus can be found in Sam Sokol, "Slammed by COVID-19, Ultra-Orthodox Jews Try to Understand What God Hath Wrought," *Times of Israel* (May 13, 2020), available at: https://www.timesofisrael.com/slammed-by-covid-19-ultra-orthodox-jews-try-to-understand-what-god-hath-wrought/.

sidious dimension of this arrogance lies not merely in its affront to God in the guise of piety but in its ultimate effect and, arguably, its purpose: to control the lives of the many believers who are searching for answers. Rather than nurturing in their disciples a degree of faith that educates them to tolerate uncertainty and still persist in their commitment to do good, they choose to deceive them with their explanations and promises that constitute a form of social control. This human effort to play God is what is considered to be idolatry![2] The same impulse drives many political leaders to propose their science-defying diagnoses and cures for Covid-19 and then to impose their self-serving policies with a certitude and finality whose intention is to perpetuate their authority and their power.

What is called for, on the contrary, in the face of uncertainty and a natural phenomenon that has not yet been mastered is a profound sense of humility. This is an "I don't know" moment; we are, after all, only human. And that is, in fact, one of the more insightful understandings of the impact of God on our circumstances and our egos. The deeper significance of our affirmation of God is that as mortals we simply don't know everything and must struggle to gain as much knowledge as possible with the realization that we can never know it all definitively.

But how does all of this square with the more traditional representation of the doctrine of "reward and punishment" which appears to ascribe specific outcomes that are consequential to certain behaviors? In the following section I will address this dilemma by first analyzing the *locus classicus* for the doctrine, Deuteronomy 11:13-21, which we recite liturgically as the second paragraph of the *Keriat Shema*, and then apply the deduced lesson to the Egyptian plague narrative.

Is This What God Hath Wrought, After All?
or What Humans Have Provoked?

In classic religious thinking, the *V'haya im shamoa*, the second paragraph of the *Shema* (Deuteronomy 11:13-21), is generally viewed as a straightforward statement of God's providential management of nature, deployed as a means of graciously rewarding obedience with appropriate rain and harvest or punishing transgression by withholding precipitation,

---

[2] Kenneth Seeskin, *No Other Gods: The Modern Struggle Against Idolatry* (West Orange, N.J.: Behrman House, 1995), 31-49.

resulting in drought, famine, and eventually, exile. This linear scheme has long troubled theologians and almost all modern Jews, especially in our post-Newtonian age. The passage couldn't really mean that if you obey God's commandments you will benefit and if you violate them you will suffer. This notion clearly defies natural law of cause and effect and presents us with an outrageous portrait of an interventionist God who manipulates nature to serve God's ends in a manner that precisely replicates the explanations posited by our contemporary rabbis for the coronavirus outbreak.

Yeshayahu Leibowitz, in his penetrating discourse on the *Shema*,[3] distinguishes between paragraph one, which outlines the religious ideal of non-contingent devotion motivated by love, and paragraph two, which delineates the religious mean, the devotional behavior of the average religionist which is activated either by an expectation of a divine response/reward or by a fear of God's punishment. The first mode is described as *lishma*, for its own sake, because it was commanded and is right, whereas the second posture is termed *shelo lishma*, conditional, for some ulterior motive. Paragraph one, *Shema*, categorically demands pure love; paragraph two, *V'haya im shamoa*, in a utilitarian voice, introduces the conditional *im*, if—"if you indeed heed" (11:13).

Why do we join these paragraphs in our prayer recitation and on the parchments in our *tefillin* and *mezuzot*, asks Leibowitz? He answers perceptively and magnanimously, emphasizing that Judaism, recognizing the elusive nature of the ideal embodied by the disciplined spiritual virtuoso, casts a wide psychological net to catch the average member of the community, who needs a religious life framed in terms of reward and punishment that can gradually propel him/her from *shelo lishma*, utilitarian observance, toward *lishma*, pure devotion. The tradition is being educationally sensitive and communally inclusive. Not only do all have a place in the dynamic continuum of Judaism, but implicit is an awareness that even the elite cannot always maintain their perfect stance.

This approach—which grounds reward and punishment in the context of the contrast between utilitarian and non-contingent worship (*shelo lishma* and *lishma*)—is most emphatically articulated by Maimonides in the

---

[3] Yeshayahu Leibowitz, "Parshat Ekev," *Seven Years of Discourses on the Weekly Torah Reading* (Jerusalem: Keter, 2000), 797-802 (Hebrew).

Guide of the Perplexed,[4] in his Introduction to *Helek*,[5] and in the *Mishneh Torah*.[6] He presents the doctrine itself as an educational artifice intended to entice and train the young and untutored to develop the capacity for emotional and intellectual "indifference" in their devotion. The process involves shifting from a fear-based religiosity to one motivated by pure love, as would be the ideal love between people. The most elevated state is achieved when one's relationship with God is not determined by, and is utterly "indifferent" to, the vagaries of fate, be they beautifully grand or harshly devastating. One of the goals of education is to move the student along the continuum, away from a childish attitude that conditions his/her commitment on receiving some perceptible payoff. As Maimonides writes, "Therefore, when one teaches children, one should instruct them to serve out of fear and in order to receive reward until they mature and become much wiser. Then, one will reveal *this secret* to them slowly and accustom them to this matter gently, until they understand it and know it and serve out of love."[7] What is the secret to which he alludes? Is it possibly that there really is no reward and punishment and that genuine worship can only be unconditional? All other efforts, from his perspective, appear to constitute, at best, preparation for the authentic, love-driven religious act.[8] The goal is to outgrow the puerile dependency and to realize that a simplistic reading of *V'haya* ... is theologically wanting. Only then will a person be primed to fully appreciate the profound warning linking human behavior to natural occurrences that is imparted in the paragraph, as explicated in the following section.

The Confluence of the Natural Order and Human Morality: *We Are One*

As to the explicit linkage in Deuteronomy 11 between nature's bounty and human compliance, I would like to suggest that the relationship is not

---

[4] III:27-28.

[5] Moses Maimonides, *Commentary on the Mishnah, Order of Nezikin*, ed. Joseph Kafah (Jerusalem: Mossad Harav Kook, 1963-1968), 134-136.

[6] Teshuva ch. 10.

[7] Ibid. 10:5 (emphasis mine).

[8] This may be a clear example of the distinction that Maimonides draws, in the *Guide* III:28, between the correct belief, "which is the one and only thing aimed at," and a necessary belief, "for the acquisition of a noble moral quality."

at all outlandish. Let's first interpret the *mitzvah* observance mandated by the text more broadly to represent the moral life envisaged by scriptural teaching as a desideratum (*mitzvah*) and rain and harvest to symbolize the climatic and environmental aspects of nature. If so, the passage could serve as a warning to maintain a morally harmonious life guided by principled interaction with our fellow humans and surroundings (positive commandments) as well as limiting restraints (negative commandments), lest an abusive disequilibrium result in a catastrophic natural disaster. Although the language of biblical transmission is thoroughly theological, attributing the response to human actions directly to God, I prefer an anthropocentric interpretation that locates the flow of cause and effect solely in the human realm. Nature's bounteous yields and calamities are not to be narrowly viewed as divine rewards and punishments expressing God's beneficence and anger, but as the consequence of deliberate human endeavors. It's not that *we* cause the rain to fall, nor is it simply that our agricultural policies affect fertility and productivity. The Bible is making a complex moral case for the impact of human attitudes and behaviors toward God and our fellow humans on the earth itself. When society is in disarray; when God's word no longer shapes and limits our choices; in short, when we become abusive in our interactions, nature will respond in kind.

The agricultural Torah of antiquity envisions an ecosystem in which all of creation is interrelated and in which it is our task to mold a harmonious interplay between the various extant forces. This means that it is not only our natural undertakings, e.g., planting policies, crop rotation, land conservation, etc., that have an impact on the earth and its productivity, but social mores and even religious devotion as well. We humans are intimately connected to our surroundings and what we do, day to day, reverberates through all of creation. We are literally one! As Joseph ibn Kaspi, medieval Jewish philosopher and exegete, writes, "In our pride we foolishly imagine that there is no kinship between us and the rest of the animal world, how much less with plants and minerals... The Torah inculcates in us a sense of our modesty and lowliness, that we should even be cognizant of the fact that we are of the same stuff as the ass and the mule, the cabbage and the pomegranate and even the lifeless stone... We and the vegetables like the cabbage and the lettuce are brothers, sharing one father."[9]

Thus, the "reward and punishment" of Deuteronomy 11 is freed from its God-dominating scaffolding and transferred into a broad human-environmental framework. The lesson is that our behavior counts and that it has consequences beyond you and me. It affects nature itself.[10] This insight has now opened a new window through which to view the Egyptian plague narrative in Exodus.

"Der Mentsh Tracht un Got Lacht" (Humans Plan and God Laughs)

From the outset the biblical text makes it clear that the plagues are intended to demonstrate to Pharaoh and the Egyptians that the God of Israel, YHWH, is the Master. In response to Pharaoh's challenge, "Who is YHWH that I should heed him?" (Exodus 5:2), God declares: "But I will harden Pharaoh's heart, that I may multiply My signs and wonders in the land of Egypt. When Pharaoh does not heed you, I will lay My hand upon Egypt and deliver My battalions, My people the Israelites, from the land of Egypt with great retributions. **And the Egyptians should know that I am YHWH (the Lord), when I stretch out My hand over Egypt and bring out the Israelites from their midst**" (Exodus 7:3-5). In my reconstructed dialogue, Pharaoh, who is perceived to be divine by his subjects, a god in his own eyes,[11] tells Moses, "I know all the gods. I have scrolls that list by name all the gods of the universe. But your God appears nowhere; there is no record of Him." God then responds, "If that is the case then this is all-out war," as it says, "And I will mete out punishments to all the gods of Egypt, I YHWH" (Exodus 12:12).

A hint that the tradition is aware of the associative connection between the "gods" and the "plagues" is found in Rashi's comment to Exodus 10:10, "See that *ra'ah* (evil) is set against you."[12] Rashi comments, "I have heard a *Midrashic* explanation that there is a star by the name of *ra'ah* (evil)." *Ra'ah*

---

[9] Joseph ibn Kaspi, *Matzref la-Kesef* (Krakow: Joseph Fischer, 1906), 293-294, and *Tirat Kesef* (Pressburg: Abraham Alkalai and Son, 1905), 35-36.

[10] See Abraham Isaac ha-Kohen Kook, *Orot ha-kodesh*, vol. 3 (Jerusalem: Mossad Harav Kook, 1964), pp.64-5, "The Torah of Israel explains how the continued existence of the world and human morality are dependent on one another." Human immorality, according to Rav Kook, results in "the world rebelling against us."

[11] See *Exodus Rabbah* 5:14, "For I am the Lord of the Universe and I have created myself and the Nile."

[12] Rashi, Exodus 10:10.

is being linked by Rashi to a natural force. Cassuto then adds, "We may see here a hint to the Egyptian god *Ra*, the sun, the chief of the pantheon."[13] This means that Pharaoh was issuing a warning: "Know that the power of my god will rise against you" (so, too, 5:19 and 32:12). A fundamental principle of the pagan worldview was that if you controlled nature then you were a god. Pharaoh was identified with *Ra*, the sun god. And he, like many "Sun Kings" after him who claimed divinity, arrogated to himself a sense of dominance and superiority over all. He was the lord, the embodiment of the evil star that YHWH intended to extinguish.

Herein can be found clear evidence that the articulated purpose of the plagues was to humiliate and rout Pharaoh and the Egyptian gods. The punishment for the subjugation and oppression of Israel is utter defeat. It is represented as a war to the finish between the invisible God of history and morality who has a covenantal relationship with the descendants of the loyal and righteous Patriarchs of Israel and the powerful nature gods of Egypt and the entire ancient world. Each of the plagues, in particular, is directed against another of the Egyptian deities, e.g., Nile turned to blood—Knum: guardian of the Nile; frogs—Heqt: god of resurrection; *dever* (plague on cattle)—Hat'hor: mother-goddess in the form of a cow; locusts—Seth: protector of crops; darkness—Ra, Atum, Horus: all sun gods; death of firstborn—Osiris: the deity of Pharaoh, the giver of life. In this way the entire sojourn in and liberation from Egypt serve as a monotheistic polemic against paganism giving definition to Israel's mission. This minor and insignificant people, Israel, is to take the world stage as the "dragon slayers," the destroyers of the mightiest and wealthiest empire in antiquity, so as to establish the credentials of their redeeming God and continue thenceforth through their prophets to spread the monotheistic message that will ultimately bring freedom to humanity. Egypt is the staging ground for Israel's revolutionary vocation.

All of the above, however, reflects only a surface reading of the narrative. On a deeper level the text hints at an even more profound lesson that is consonant with my theory of human cause and effect.

Ziony Zevit, a distinguished scholar of the Ancient Near East and a Professor of Bible at the American Jewish University, has published a

---

[13] Umberto Cassuto, *A Commentary on the Book of Exodus*, trans. Israel Abrahams (Jerusalem: Magnes Press, 1967), Exodus 10:10.

series of illuminating articles regarding the plagues.[14] The novelty in his approach is his focus on the linguistic connections between the plague cycle in Exodus and the creation passage in Genesis or, more pointedly, on the invocation of creation in the story of the ten plagues. A few examples will suffice: 1. The Hebrew word used for the Egyptian gatherings of water, in God's instruction regarding the initiation of the blood plague, is *mikveh* (Exodus 7:19). This is the same term used in Genesis 1:10—"God called the dry land earth and the *mikveh* (gatherings) of water God called Seas"; 2. When it comes to frogs, their emergence from the Nile is described as swarming—"The Nile shall swarm *(sharatz)* with frogs" (Exodus 7:28). This is the same rare biblical verb used in Genesis 1:20, "Let the waters bring forth *(yishretzu)* swarms of living creatures"; and 3. There is a glaring contrast between the generative creation on day three—"The land brought forth vegetation: seed bearing fruit with seed in it" (Genesis 1:12)—and Exodus 10:15 where in the aftermath of the locust plague "nothing green was left of tree or grass of the field in all the land of Egypt."

Most significantly, the darkness "that can be touched" (Exodus 10:21) signifies the cessation of the alternation of light and darkness, of day and night, and the total disappearance of the sun. Egypt was thereby thrust into a pre-creation mode of existence. Finally, the death of the firstborn represents the complete reversal of the crowning act of creation: human life itself is destroyed—initially only the firstborn, but then at the sea the glory of Egypt, its cavalry and Pharaoh himself, is swallowed up and consumed. Egypt's life-force is no more!

What is obvious is that the plagues progress in a process that unleashes affliction after affliction leading to a cataclysmic crescendo that concludes with the absolute undoing of creation. Egyptian reality is overturned as that exceedingly ordered and regimented society devolves into a state of chaos. Nature is turned against itself and is no longer fruitful and life-giving. Let us not forget that the Nile, the life-sustaining "god" of Egypt, in an overture to the devastation that follows, is turned into blood, a graphic symbol of death. Creation is reversed and life is transmuted into death.

---

[14] Ziony Zevit, "The Priestly Redaction and Interpretation of the Plague Narrative in Exodus," *Jewish Quarterly Review* 66:4 (April 1976): 193-211; idem, "Three Ways to Look at the Ten Plagues," *Bible Review* 6:3 (June 1990): 16-23, 42; idem, "The Ten Plagues and Egyptian Ecology," *TheTorah.com* (January 9, 2015); idem, "Invoking Creation in the Story of the Ten Plagues," *TheTorah.com* (March 25, 2015).

As if to further emphasize this point, the aggregation of a ten-plague cycle corresponds to the "ten divine utterances by which the world was created" (*Avot* 5:1). Ten plagues strike Egypt so as to undo the world that God created with ten utterances. And in the wake of the fall of Egypt, Israel rises, forged out of the chaos. This, too, is conveyed symbolically when God bestows ten commandments upon Israel in a redemptive encounter that is intended to repair the creation that has been unraveled through ten plagues.[15]

Essential to maintaining a productive environment, then, is living with a God-fearing discipline (*mitzvot*) and recognizing the One who is beyond all gods, all humans, all Pharaohs. This idea is exquisitely represented by the Shabbat whose required observance, situated at the heart of the ten commandments, resonates with the two themes of creation and exodus found in the two versions of the ten commandments (Exodus 20:8-11, Deuteronomy 5:12-15). They are then inscribed in the hearts and minds of all Jews through the Friday night *Kiddush* recitation that incorporates a reference to both.[16] The Exodus, thus understood, constitutes a new creation: the creation of God's people, Israel.

An inference to be drawn from the symbolic linkage established between the propitious promise of creation and the overturning of the Egyptian order as a response to pharaonic persecution is that the "miraculous" episode being portrayed in the text need not be taken literally. Rather, the narrative depicting a mythic confrontation between YHWH and the gods is a transparent screen that artfully communicates the dynamic struggle between two moral-religious worldviews: the one propelled by power, authority, and dominance that I'll call "the arrogance of power" and the other driven by covenantal commitment, compassion, and devotion that I'll call "devotional humility." Pharaoh projects "the arrogance of power," whereas Moses and YHWH introduce "devotional humility." The story cycle of warning and punishment by debilitating pestilence is not at all a historical account of God's mighty hand striking Egypt again and again but really the tragic report of self-inflicted chaos and destruction. Pharaoh's

---

[15] Cf. *Pesikta Rabbati* 21; *Zohar* 3:11b-12a; Abraham Saba, *Tzeror ha-Mor* (Bnei Brak: Heichal ha-Sefer, 1990), 373-375; Judah Aryeh Leib Alter, *Sefat Emet* (Merkaz Shapira: Yeshivat Or Etzion, 2001), *Yitro* 1893, s.v. *mitzvat*.

[16] See the *Koren-Sacks Siddur* (Jerusalem: Koren Publishers Jerusalem Ltd., 2009), 382-383.

treatment of his Israelite subjects reaches levels of inhuman abuse. His arrogance is reflected in an attitude that considers all created resources to be his to control and subdue without limits or restraints.[17]

Thus the plagues are symbolically constructed to communicate both the decimation of the Egyptian gods and of Egypt's natural order. The narrative presents a fundamental moral teaching depicting a hubristic Pharaoh who simultaneously abuses his human subjects and his environment, occasioning the collapse of the Egyptian Empire itself. Redemption comes to those who humbly devote themselves to the "One who is beyond all."

Pharaoh had set himself up as the personification of "god," the final arbiter and ruler of the universe. This is the key to understanding why it is that the Bible is so determined to eradicate paganism. What is the great offense that is involved? It is none but the ultimate idolatry of self-deification: one human who uses and abuses all creatures, all humans and all of creation to such an extent that he wreaks havoc with his world and, unable to heed the warning signs (plagues), gradually self-destructs in a convulsive collapse. This is the saga repeatedly endured by every empire since time immemorial. Empires eventually eat themselves up, consumed by their own collective pridefulness and the uncontained hubris of their leaders. This pattern persists to our own day with one example after another of the inevitable implosion of a seemingly invincible superpower and its pharaonic overlord. The biblical God, on the contrary, is life-giving and sustaining, creating human partners with freedom, agency and responsibility.

The big idea in this interpretation is that just as in Deuteronomy 11 human morality affects nature, so, too, in Egypt it is Pharaoh's disregard for and claim of mastery over fellow human beings, which is inexorably tied to his rapacious misuse of resources, that occasions the onslaught of the plagues. His penchant for constructing grand monuments reflects a nature-controlling and -defying outlook that manifests in a whole range of priestly rituals and public displays demonstrating Pharaoh's claim of eternity. Everything and everyone is at Pharaoh's disposal—literally, no stone can be left unturned—in his pursuit of the "elixir of immortality." The moral message of the first slave revolution in recorded history, that

---

[17] See Ezekiel 29:3, "My Nile is mine, and I made it for myself," and *Exodus Rabbah* 5:14 and 8:2.

no human has the right to subjugate another, is paralleled in the natural domain by the principle that no human is the absolute master of the environment. In time, nature that is trampled and violated rebels just as does suppressed human nature.

A Lesson for Our Time

An instructive and insightful depiction of the lived consequence of life under an oppressive regime that abuses both its human subjects and its natural resources was introduced in the Tanner Lecture presented to an overflow crowd in UCLA's Royce Hall on October 25, 1991 by Václav Havel, the President of the Czech and Slovak Federal Republic. Havel explained:

> The Communist rulers of Czechoslovakia operated according to the all-or-nothing principle of *"après nous le déluge."* Hoping that no one would notice, they secured absolute power by bribing the entire population with money stolen from future generations. Miners extracting low-quality brown coal from strip mines—coal that was then burned without filters—were grateful for the chance to buy VCRs, and exhausted after a day's work, eyes glued to the screen, they failed to notice the pus flowing from the eyes of their children. Their wives noticed... *Après nous le déluge* is the principle of a person who is related to no order but that of his own benefit; it is the nihilistic principle of a person who has forgotten he is but a part of the world and not its owner, of a person who feels no relation to eternity and styles himself master of space and time.

> I believe that the devastation of the environment brought about by the Communist regime is a warning to all contemporary civilization. I believe you should read the message coming from our part of the world as an appeal against all those who despise the mystery of being, whether they be cynical businessmen with only the interests of their corporations at heart or left-wing saviors high on cheap ideological utopias. Both lack something I would call a metaphysical anchor, that is,

a humble respect for the whole of creation and a consciousness of our obligation to it.

Were I to encapsulate the experience in one sentence, I would formulate it as follows: If parents believe in God, their children will not need to wear gas masks to school and their children's eyes will be free of pus.[18]

The Communists, according to Havel, had no ecological sensibility, no regard for the environment and its resources. Concomitantly, they had no regard for individual human life. The goal was to maximize industrial productivity at all costs. In the process they transformed Poland from Europe's breadbasket to its basket-case and polluted the Czech environment to the detriment of tens of thousands. The abuse of resources went hand-in-hand with the abuse of human beings. It involved total indifference to the natural ecosystem that relied upon rational-moral policies reflecting human respect for nature and governmental respect for human beings. Like the Pharaohs of old, the Communists had absolute control and authority and there were no limits, no restraints, on what they intended to achieve using the raw materials at their disposal. And indeed, the people, much like the material resources, were all disposable and replaceable. Their worldview was guided by "the arrogance of power." Humility was nowhere. As Abraham had declared in defending his case to Abimelech, "I thought, surely, there is no fear of God in this place" (Genesis 20:11). The absence of *yirat Elohim*—the fear of God—is the consistent driving force behind the Bible's struggle against idolatry. Every power-revering government in history has invariably oppressed its citizens and despoiled its resources—which brings us back to our Corona plague.

It is no accident that the virus originated in and emanated from China. It, too, is a Communist society where rulers, time after time, have demonstrated no respect for the individual lives of their citizens and no regard for their natural resources. It's all about economic growth and material success, what they term the "China miracle." No humility here; rather, total control. And there are no limits on use and abuse. Whether it's the

---

[18] The Tanner Lecture delivered by Václav Havel, President of the Czech and Slovak Federal Republic, at UCLA, October 25, 1991.

consumption of every species of wildlife, including those that are the carriers of unknown viral strains, or the disastrous damming of its main waterway, everything is at play. Most egregious of all, Chinese officials chose to suppress the initial reports of the coronavirus and subsequently failed to sound a timely alarm to world health officials because they didn't want "to look bad." The main priority was and is commerce, trade, profit, and power. Human well-being is secondary. And so China floods the market with inferior and dangerous drugs, faulty machines and harmful toys. They don't care; there is no place for caring.

The troubling question is: has this same lack of humility in the form of governmental arrogance and a broad-based culture of greed seeped into our democratic institutions in the United States and corroded our own founding principle of "We the People"? How often have we heard, "I'm in control," "look at the soaring economy," the "greatest"? Contrast this with the constructive humility of the truly great: Washington and Lincoln. How sad that the same consideration operative in China, fear of appearing "to look bad," has been echoed in our own precincts, as well. Just as with the Chinese, saving face has become more vital than saving lives. Have our values been distorted and our systems corrupted to the extent that life and nature have been objectively commodified in an unrelenting, "idolatrous" pursuit of more?

All around us nature is signaling that our unlimited expansion and infringement endangers the endurance of our civilization. We desperately need a reboot and a repair that will motivate us to transform our "culture of greed" into a "culture of enough." Then, in addition to the essential "herd immunity," we will have an opportunity to engender the equally crucial "herd humility and decency." Only then will we have a chance at establishing the Abrahamic standard of *yirat Elohim* in this place. It is the key to our survival and to our renewal.

Love in a Time of Absence: Reading Rashi's Song of Songs Commentary During Coronavirus

Devorah Schoenfeld

A global pandemic is experienced by everyone together; and at the same time, everyone's experience of it is unique. For me so much of the experience has been about isolation, about absence from community and from people I love. In times of absence and isolation the question of how to love God can feel very important. With the synagogues closed and so many of the Jewish community experiencing *Shabbatot* and holidays on our own, we are cut off from many ways we normally experience our relationship with God. So, how do we love God in this present circumstance? How do we talk about and understand love of God—no matter how alone we might feel and no matter what pain we might be experiencing?

In thinking about love of God, one place to turn to is the interpretation of Song of Songs, because that is one place that Jewish exegetes think about love between God and Israel. Although the Song of Songs is often read as a single, continuous story, it has in it elements of both unity and multiplicity. It has consistent imagery, themes and style, but the protagonists and settings shift. Because of this, some scholars have read it as a unified text, while others have read it as a collection.[1] When we recognize the multiplicity in the Song of Songs, it can become a book about how different kinds of love of God are possible and sacred.[2]

In this article I will read not the Song of Songs itself, but the commentary of Rashi (1040-1106) on it, and look at the different models it presents of how to love God when God is absent. Rashi's commentary on the entire Tanakh was extremely influential on Jewish readings of the Bible, and his

---

[1] For an overview of the problem, see Marc Brettler, "Unresolved and Unresolvable Problems in Interpreting the Song" in Peter S. Hawkins, Lesleigh Cushing Stahlberg, eds. *Scrolls of Love: Reading Ruth and the Song of Songs* (New York: Fordham University Press, 2006).

[2] My forthcoming book, *How Many Lovers Are In the Song of Songs? The Unity and Multiplicity of the Song of Songs in Historical and Theological Perspectives,* will examine the theological implications of the multiple characters and settings of the Song of Songs as they have been interpreted by classical and medieval exegetes.

Song of Songs commentary is a model for how the book continues to be read by many in the Jewish community today. Rashi, writing in twelfth-century France, followed the tradition of reading Song of Songs as an allegory for the love between God and Israel.[3] He drew on midrashic interpretations of Song of Songs and wove them together to tell a story about a woman longing for her estranged husband, which is at the same time a story of God's love for Israel:

> And this book is based, by the holy spirit, in the metaphor of a woman bound in living widowhood (2 Sam. 20.3), longing for her husband, leaning on her beloved, remembering the love of her youth for him and admitting her sins. Her beloved is also suffering with her in her pain (Isaiah 63.9), and remembers the love of her youth and the beauty of her beauty, and the rightness of her deeds, that with them he was connected with her in a powerful love, so that she might know that he is not causing her suffering from his heart (Lamentations 3.33) and she has not truly been divorced (Isaiah 50.1), for she is still his wife and he her husband (Hosea 2.4) and he will return to her.[4]

Rashi tells here a story of a woman who is suffering because her husband has abandoned but not divorced her, and how, despite their mutual estrangement, they still long for each other. At the same time, Song of Songs is also about the relationship between God and Israel, in which Israel reflects on its relationship with God while in exile. These two stories, for Rashi, take place at the same time in the same text. So Rashi constructs two different narratives out of a conviction that the text can hold a multiplicity of meaning, a conviction that he states through the two quotations with which he begins his introduction:

---

[3] Classical and medieval Jewish exegetes typically either read the Song of Songs as about God's love for Israel or, as Rashi does, as operating on two levels: a love story between two people and a love story between Israel and God. For an in-depth study of Jewish Song of Songs exegesis see Michael Fishbane, *The JPS Bible Commentary: Song of Songs*, (Philadelphia: The Jewish Publication Society, 2015).

[4] Rashi's introduction to Song of Songs. All translations are my own, with verse citations added for the convenience of the reader. The text of Rashi that I am using is from *Mikraot Gedolot Haketer* [Hebrew], ed. Menachem Cohen (Ramat Gan: Bar Ilan University, 2012).

God said one thing, I heard two. (Psalms 62:12).

One text brings forth multiple meanings (Sanhedrin 34a).[5]

Rashi weaves together the different songs in Song of Songs and their different midrashic interpretations by framing them through four characters: wife and husband, Israel and God. The multiplicity of the original text, however, still comes through in the way Rashi separates these songs into different monologues and dialogues, each with their own setting and theme. Some of the individual songs in the Song of Songs are in the wife's voice, some are in her husband's, and others are a conversation between them. The songs that describe the absence of the husband from the wife, or God from Israel, describe the meaning of that separation in different ways and connect it to different biblical stories. The variety of approaches to God's absence in Rashi's Song of Songs commentary allows for the recognition that there is no one way to love God and no single response to absence or tragedy. It allows for the different ways we experience this pandemic that we are all going through together.

The monologues in which the husband and wife are separated deal with the theme of absence in different ways. They are distinct, and each connects to different biblical stories and draws on different possible theological meanings for the separation. In his comments on different monologues, Rashi offers several ways to imagine Israel loving God in God's absence.

Song of Songs 1:2-4—Love remembers

Song of Songs 1:2-4 is a song about someone longing for kisses from a lover who is a king. The speaker asks to follow the king into the king's chambers. In Rashi's commentary on these verses, they are in the voice of the estranged wife who is thinking about her estranged husband, missing him and wishing he would return. At the same time, it is also in the voice of Israel thinking about God while in exile. Writing in exile, Israel remembers when God saved them from Egypt. The memory of the past redemption holds the key to future redemption.

Rashi shows us how memory and storytelling can work through two

---

[5] Rashi's introduction to Song of Songs.

figures who appear here, Rahab and Jethro:

> "This is why young women love you." (Song of Songs 1:3) Jethro came when he heard the news and converted. Also Rahab the prostitute said, "We heard how God dried up [the Red Sea]"(Joshua 2:10) and because of this she said "The LORD your God is God in heaven" (Joshua 2:11).[6]

Rahab and Jethro are important in Rashi's story because the story of the Exodus, rather than its lived memory, is what brings them closer to God. Both are, according to Rashi, non-Jews who converted to Judaism after hearing how God saved the Israelites from Egypt.[7]

The story of these converts is important here because it shows that the path to union with God is always possible, and here what makes it possible is the story of what happened in the past, whether or not one personally remembers it. Rahab and Jethro were not present at the Exodus, but the story of it helps them come closer to God. So, too, what makes Israel's return to God possible is the retelling of the story of the Exodus, even when those retelling the story of the Exodus did not experience it themselves. This is the first solution that Rashi gives for dealing with the problem of Divine absence: tell stories of when things were better.

Song of Songs 4:6-8—Love is always present

Song of Songs 4:6-8 tells a very different story from the previous one. In it, the two protagonists can only be together for a short time, until the sun is hottest, and then they will have to go. The man asks the woman to come with him to different places: Lebanon, the peak of Amanah, lion's dens.

In Rashi's story about God and Israel, this is God saying to Israel: Eventually you will be exiled from the Temple. And when that happens:

> "Come with me from Lebanon, Bride." (Song of Songs 4:8)

---

[6] Rashi on Song of Songs 1:2-4.

[7] In Rashi's commentary to Exodus 18:1 he explains that Jethro came to join Moses and the Israelites as a convert after hearing about the exodus. According to Megillah 14b, Rahab converted and married Joshua.

When you are exiled from this Lebanon you will be exiled
with me, because I will be exiled with you. [8]

God promises to go with Israel into exile. God continues the promise:

And when you return from exile, I will return with you, and
also all the days of the exile, I will suffer when you do.[9]

God promises to be with Israel wherever they are, whether in exile
or returned from exile. God further promises to not only be with Israel
physically but also to be with Israel emotionally—to be present in Israel's
suffering.

In explaining this verse, Rashi connects it to a different biblical story
in which God was with someone who was distressed: the story of the end
of the life of Moses.

Another explanation, "From the peak of Amanah" (Song of
Songs 4:8), this mountain on the northern boundary of the
Land of Israel is called Amanah. In the Mishnah (Gittin 8a)
it is called Amnon and is Mount Hor, about which is said,
"from the Great Sea you shall draw a line from the Great Sea to
Mount Hor" (Numbers 34:7). When the exiles together reach
there, they will look from there and see the air of the land of
Israel and they will be happy and sing in praise.[10]

In this explanation, Rashi connects this story of God being with Israel
in exile to Moses describing the borders to the Israelites before they cross
over the Jordan—to go into the land of Israel without him. Moses dies
in exile and will not himself go into the land that he is describing. But
Moses died with God's kiss: even though he never personally returned
from exile, God was still with him. So, too, Rashi says, God is with all
the generations of Israel, those who will return and those who will only
see the land from a distance. According to Rashi, Moses describing the

---

[8] Rashi on Song of Songs 4.8.
[9] Rashi on Song of Songs 4:8.
[10] Rashi on Song of Songs 4:8.

borders of Israel from the desert is his thinking about the praise that future generations will sing.

In this second approach, Rashi calls on those who love God in a time of exile to find God where they are, and to feel God's love where they are—even in troubling times, even in exile. Both Israel and God commit to a future in which they are together, in all the places they will go. God might seem to be absent but in reality is always present.

Song of Songs 5:2-7—Love accepts rebuke

Chapter 5 verses 2-7 of Song of Songs tells yet another very different story, of a woman whose lover comes to her at night. She hesitates to open the door for him; when she does, he is gone. She goes out in search of him and instead finds guards who beat and abuse her. The woman here has done wrong, which she acknowledges, in not opening the door for her lover. At the same time, she is caught in a situation of injustice where the guards attack her and beat her unprovoked.

Rashi here interprets the woman as not wanting to open the door for her husband because she is committing adultery. In his observation of Song of Songs 5:3, he writes, "The expression, 'I have taken off my cloak ... I have washed my feet' is the answer of an adulterous wife, who does not want to open the door for her husband."[11] In Rashi's theological interpretation, this story of an adulterous wife is about Israel in the time of the First Temple, when they had the ability to be with God and God wanted to be with them. But Israel hesitated to seek God, and was not able to fully renounce idolatry. The guards who found Israel were Nebuchadnezzar and his armies that destroyed the Temple.

Rashi connects this passage to Jeremiah 44, which takes place after the destruction of Judea and Jerusalem. The few Judeans left in Judah had fled to Egypt and had taken Jeremiah with them, even though Jeremiah had prophesied that God wanted them to stay in Judea. In this passage, Jeremiah asks the Judeans living in Egypt to return to God and turn away from idolatry, explaining that everything bad that has happened to them has been because of their turning away from God. They tell Jeremiah that they will continue to worship the Queen of Heaven because when they

---

[11] Rashi on Song of Songs 5:3.

did things were better:

> We will not do the thing that you said that we should do in the name of the LORD. Rather, we will do what we have said we will do. We will make offerings to the Queen of Heaven and to pour libations to her, like we and our fathers, our kings and our officials used to do in the towns of Judah and the streets of Jerusalem, and were sated with bread and it was good for us and we never saw anything bad.[12]

These Judeans are continuing to engage in idolatry even though they are experiencing God's punishment for doing so. They remember the distant past when idolatry worked well for them and want to go back to that past rather than recognize that God is punishing them for idolatry in the present.

In this third approach of Rashi's to understanding exile, distance from God is a consequence of collective and individual rejection of God. The personal betrayal of the woman who will not open the door because she is engaged in adultery is parallel to that of the collective group who are not willing to stop their idolatry. Idolatry here may be nothing more than unwillingness to change old practices or to listen to a rebuke.

At the same time there are other people causing harm that the protagonists might not be able to stop. The wife may be committing adultery, but she is still being cruelly harmed by the city guards. Similarly, the Judeans may be persisting in idolatry, but Nebuchadnezzar and his armies are still coming to exile them.

This third approach asks us to love God by asking whether we are remaining faithful to God's love, and by demanding that we make changes if we are not. In the same way, some of us are looking at our own individual choices and asking if we are taking the necessary steps to protect our own and one another's lives. Some of us are also looking outward, asking whether the country we are in is doing the necessary work to protect the lives of all those in it; or if, like the guards in this song, it is instead harming them. This approach asks us to use this time of absence to accept rebuke and to reflect on what we can do better—as individuals and

---

[12] Jeremiah 44:16-17.

as a community.

Song of Songs 8:2-3—Love returns

Song of Songs ends in Chapter 8 with a song of the female protagonist yearning and hoping for reunion with her beloved. She wishes that her beloved were her brother so that she could kiss him in public and bring him home to her mother's house. To Rashi, this is also a story of Israel yearning for God to comfort them in exile. Rashi compares this yearning to the story of Joseph:

> **If only you were like a brother to me.** That you would come and comfort me like Joseph did to for brothers who wronged him, and it is said "he comforted them" (Genesis 50:21).[13]

The story of Joseph comforting his brothers is one of the most classic examples of something that looks like a tragedy turning out for the best. As Joseph explains to his brothers:

> Now do not be sad and do not be angry with yourselves because you sold me here, because God sent me here to preserve life. The famine has been here for two years and there will not be plowing or harvest for another five. God sent me ahead of you to ensure that you survive on earth and to save your lives in a great deliverance. Therefore, it was not you who sent me here but God, who made me like a father to Pharaoh, as lord of all his household, and ruler over the whole land of Egypt.[14]

Joseph was able to reorganize Egyptian society in a way that prevented deaths from famine. His brothers were able to show that they had changed; when Joseph asked them to abandon Benjamin as they had abandoned Joseph himself, they refused. Joseph's brothers were willing to act ethically and responsibly and Joseph was willing to forgive them. After all this, in retrospect, Joseph was able to see everything that happened to him as an

---

[13] Rashi on Song of Songs 8:1.
[14] Genesis 45:5-8.

act of God in which God was present and engaged.

The story of Joseph is one of the last stories that Rashi cites in his Song of Songs commentary, and the Exodus is one of the first. But because in the Torah itself the story of Joseph leads into the story of the Exodus, the story of the Song of Songs in Rashi is cyclical as well as linear. The Jewish people's history moves linearly, from Abraham, through Joseph, through Moses and the Exodus, to exile and the hope of a future return. But it also moves in cycles, from distance from God to closeness with God and back again. The classic statement of this cycle is from Deuteronomy:

> I call heaven and earth this day to witness against you that you will certainly be gone from the land that you are crossing the Jordan to inherit, you will not have long days there but will be destroyed. The LORD will disperse you among the nations, and only a small number of you will be left among the nations to which the LORD will send you. There you will serve gods that people have made from wood and stone, that do not see or hear or eat or smell. And you will seek from there for the LORD your God and you will find, if you seek Him with all your heart and soul when you are suffering because all that you have found, and return to God and listen to His voice. (Deut. 4:26-30)

These verses describe a cycle in which sin is followed by exile, which is followed by repentance, which is in turn followed by return from exile. This cycle of sin and repentance, exile and return will be enacted, and repeated over and over, through the stories in Joshua, Samuel, and the two books of Kings.

This fourth approach suggests that tragedy and distance from God are part of a cycle that can lead to things becoming better in a way that depends on our own choices. Reading it in coronavirus times, it asks what we can change so that the cycle can move forward. Is there anything good that can come to us from this tragedy of Covid-19 and the compounding tragedy of a governmental response that has made things worse?

Conclusion: Love hopes

In the last song in the Song of Songs, a woman sitting in a garden calls on her lover while her friends listen, and asks him to come to her, "like a young hart or a gazelle" (Song of Songs 8:14). Rashi sees this as Israel yearning for redemption. In his commentary on the previous verse, Israel in exile calls on God:

> **The one who sits in the gardens.** The Holy Blessed One says to the community of Israel, "You are dispersed in exile, grazing in the gardens of others but sitting in synagogues and study halls."[15]

For Rashi, this describes the present reality where Israel is in exile and scattered, but engaged in prayer and study. When she calls on God to come to her, in the words of Rashi, she is asking God to hasten the future redemption:

> **Flee, beloved.** From exile and redeem us from among them.

> **And be like a gazelle**. To bring redemption quickly, and to bring Your Divine Presence to rest **upon the mountains of spices**. This is Mount Moriah and the Holy Temple, may it be rebuilt speedily and in our days, Amen.[16]

In this conclusion, Rashi invites the Jewish people to call on God to end the exile.

Rashi's commentary on Song of Songs offers us many ways of coming to terms with Divine absence and exile. We can tell stories of past redemptions and find hope in them. We can recognize God's presence in the exile itself. We can recognize the wrongs that we have done to cause distance from God. We can find good in everything that has come about. But ultimately, Rashi writes, one should not become too accustomed to

---

[15] Rashi on Song of Songs 8:13.
[16] Rashi on Song of Songs 8:14.

Divine absence. Although the Song of Songs ends, in Rashi's reading, with Israel still in exile, it also concludes with Israel expressing hope for return.

Reading this in times of suffering, isolated from family, community and synagogue, in a country in which the effects of the pandemic are felt disproportionately by those already marginalized, it is easy to imagine that what has gone wrong can never be fixed. Rashi issues a demand that we not do that. In the end, Israel still asks God to return to her and with her. In the end, loving God means continuing to have hope, remaining in the relationship and insisting on its reconstruction.

Keter and Corona: Perspectives from the Jewish Mystical Tradition

Arthur Green

Dedicated to my dear friend Melila Hellner-Eshed, co-source of some of these insights.

1

For many years I have been a student and teacher of the Jewish mystical tradition. This is a body of lore to which many have turned for healing over the centuries. They have often seen teachers of this tradition as holy people, *tzaddikim,* who have some special closeness to God, resulting in an ability to pray successfully for the healing of the sick. There is a whole realm called "practical Kabbalah," still widely practiced in Israel, both among Jews of Near Eastern origin and among *Hasidim,* that deals almost exclusively with the curative power of blessings, amulets, and holy names. Jerusalem taxicabs and market stalls are often adorned with pictures of Moroccan or Baghdadi Jewish saints or Eastern European Hasidic rabbis, showing that practical Kabbalah is alive and well among certain sectors of the Jewish community.

Over the years, various tales have come to my ears of someone who was cured from illness or saved from disaster by the blessing of the Lubavitcher or another Hasidic *rebbe.* These, of course, echoed a great deal of what was present in the mystical sources I studied. Yet I remained uninterested in—and somewhat dismissive of—the alleged curative powers of either kabbalistic amulets or the blessings of Hasidic rabbis. I considered this popular use of Kabbalah a betrayal of the deeper mystical tradition, one which saw all worship as an act of pure giving and devotion, not seeking even such reasonable earthly rewards as health and longevity.

Decades of involvement with mystical teachings do have their effect, however. I am engaged with a realm of human understanding that by definition goes beyond ordinary rules of reason or scientific explanation.

As a student of kabbalistic and Hasidic literature, I have always sought to take the mystics' testimony seriously, to analyze it on its own terms, and perhaps to compare it with language heard elsewhere, either in Jewish or non-Jewish sources. I am especially wary of reductionist or dismissive explanations. This means that I have to *listen* to the mystics of prior generations, allowing myself to becoming open to the reality they describe. I cannot cut them off when they begin describing something—a miraculous healing, for example—that my modern mind and my own life experience want to deny as absurd.

This involvement with the realm of inner mystery has forced me to admit how much there is that I—dare I say *we*—do not understand. I certainly cannot judge whether the visions or recounted experiences of mystical teachers throughout the world are "true" or not on the basis of my meager ability to explain them. I have come rather to accept them as strivings to express the ineffable, as attempts to describe an inner reality that makes powerful claims, both on the original visionaries who describe them and on later generations of faithful readers, sometimes including myself, who are inspired by them.

I have come to accept that there are forces or energies present in the world that we have not yet found ways to measure or describe. In ways we do not understand at all, there are people who have the psychic ability to "tune in" to the frequencies of these energies and come to see or know things that are otherwise beyond explanation. The field of psychic research is as yet very young and overwhelmed by both charlatanism and the excessive skepticism that comes in its wake. But I believe we still have much more to learn in this area than we know at present, and humility behooves us in our ignorance. This does not mean, of course, that we are to become patsies for the many spurious and suspicious claims in this area that appear every day.

The same has slowly come to be the case with regard to accounts of healing, whether based on the blessings of a *tzaddik*, the laying on of hands, or simply the power of prayer. As I have become aware of the defensive role that a certain cynicism about such claims plays in my own psychic life, I have been forced to become more open to the reality of experiences recounted by others.

2

There is, however, another sort of healing to be found in the study and teaching of Jewish mystical sources, one about which I have no question at all. I even consider myself a witness to its truth. This is the balm offered by beautiful teachings. The student of Zohar or of the Hasidic masters is carried on the wings of a rich symbolic language into a realm of consciousness that is inaccessible to us in our ordinary lives. The sources often refer to this experience as one of entering *heikhalot*, "palaces," but often taken as "chambers" filled with divine light. The passageway into these inner chambers is one of opening the mind, letting go of prior assumptions, and allowing oneself to fill up with an almost childlike sense of wonder.

The homilies of the Zohar, the key text of classical Kabbalah, often imitate an earlier midrashic style by beginning with "Rabbi Yehudah" or "Rabbi Hiyya *opened*..." The word *patah* there originally means "opened," as in "began." He opened his teaching with the following words. But later readers took *patah* to refer to a different sort of opening. He opened the verse to a deeper sort of reading; he used the verse as a key to open the way into those inner palaces of understanding. He opened the eyes of his readers to a realm of insight they had not previously experienced. "Reveal my eyes and I will behold wonders of Your Torah!" (Ps. 119:18).

The healing power of this engagement is difficult to describe, but entirely real. The palaces are filled with warmth and light. Basking in that light has about it some foretaste of the older rabbinic description of the afterlife, where "the righteous sit with crowns on their heads, enjoying the radiance of divine presence" (b. Berakhot 17a).

Let me take you into one of those palaces, one that comes to mind in the light of our present plague situation.

"Y-H-W-H responded to Job out of the whirlwind [*min ha-se'arah*] (Job 38:1)." The *se'arah* out of which God responded was the whirlwind of Job's life. Everything this righteous man had counted on until that moment had been upended. Health, prosperity, and family had all suddenly disappeared. All the blessings for which we pray had been taken away from him. But it was *min ha-se'arah*, from within the whirlwind itself, that Job sensed a divine response. Not an *answer*, mind you, but a *response*. The experience of the whirlwind itself was the place from which he felt this divine response. Job did not just have a *question*, something that can be answered. He stood with his entire self as a *challenge*, one that called forth the fullness of divine response, one that said: "*Hineni*; Here I am, within this whirlwind that is happening to you."

Our entire human family is living through such a whirlwind. Our most basic sense of security has been overturned. Dare I breathe the air around me? May I safely have a conversation with another human being? Is it permitted to touch? To sing? Without these, what will be left of our humanity?

We struggle in vain to look for precedents, for parallel events from which we might learn. This is not the Flood, not the Holocaust; we are not, thank God, being utterly destroyed. But there is a collective fear in the air that is entirely unfamiliar, especially for us Americans, who lack any firsthand experience with the ravages of war or plague.

The Hebrew word that comes to mind for such a moment is *shever*, "brokenness." Our ordinary understanding of how the world works—our simple confidence that we know how to survive from day to day—has been broken. *Shever* is also the root of the word *mashber*, "crisis," a time when we feel that something in our lives is deeply broken. We have become used to hearing the pandemic talked about as a health crisis, one that challenges our medical system and its ability to heal. But it is also an economic crisis, a social crisis, and so much more. It is an *existential* crisis, a threat to our very existence as we are.

Shever is used several times by the author of the biblical Lamentations— traditionally identified as the prophet Jeremiah—written in response to the destruction of Jerusalem in 587 BCE. The loss of this beautiful city called "joy of all the earth" (as it still is!) is referred to as *shever bat-ami*, the "brokenness of My daughter-people" (Lam. 4:10).)The most poignant evocation of that image comes in 2:13 of Lamentations: "How can I attest to you? To what can I liken you, O daughter of Jerusalem? To what may I compare you, to bring you comfort, virgin daughter of Zion? Your breach is as wide as the sea! Who will heal you?"

God is calling out to His beautiful city, His innocent virgin daughter. She has been raped, split open by the invading forces. The gap is "as wide as the sea," a sea so alien to landlocked Jerusalem. How could such a terrible breach ever be healed?

In comes the Zohar on its very first page (1:1b). It is not only the earthly

Jerusalem that has been so terribly invaded, but the heavenly Jerusalem, the *shekhinah*, the "daughter" within God. The old rabbinic trope of the exiled *shekhinah* ("Wherever Israel were exiled, *shekhinah* was exiled with them"), identified with Mother Rachel weeping for her children, has now been elevated into a figure of the divine feminine. The very realm of the Godhead has been breached, even raped, by the evil forces of the "Other Side," the heavenly counterpart of the earthly Babylonian armies.

"Your breach is as wide as the sea" reminds the reader that *yam*, the sea, is also a symbol-term for the *shekhinah*. The sea, like the moon, is a classic embodiment of the feminine in myth and symbol throughout literature. She is the sea into which "all the rivers flow" (Eccles. 1:7), the female divine receptacle for the flow of light, water, or seed from the mysterious beyond. Thus is the hopelessness of her situation magnified still further. She, Jerusalem, turns out to also be the sea. Of course she is breached wide open. This is her nature. Indeed, can there be any hope of healing from such a *shever*?

The Zohar's answer comes quickly, as the verse proceeds. "Who can heal you" is taken not as a question, but as a statement. The divine feminine of *shekhinah* is herself a lower manifestation of a yet deeper female force, that of *binah*, the hidden Mother of the upper worlds, the cosmic womb out of which all life flows. Because *binah* is so deeply hidden and unknowable —the way none of us can remember the womb out of which we were surely born—one of her names is *mi*, or "Who?" Thus the "Who will heal you?" of our verse turns into "The *Who* will heal you!"

How might we translate this bit of poetic hermeneutics into terms that might speak to the contemporary reader? *Shekhinah* is the divine presence to be found throughout the world. But the world around us indeed seems deeply broken. We hesitate before going out of doors, especially in the city, lest we be pounced upon by some mysterious droplets left over from an anonymous passerby's cough. How thoroughly polluted that outer realm seems to be. This is the brokenness amidst which we find ourselves, as soon as we step out the door. But there is an answer. Go deeper—turn to a more secret inner place, one that you have to traverse forty-nine intricate pathways to reach. Those pathways are all the complex inter-weavings of deed and emotion that constitute your religious life, your pathways of walking through the world. But when you direct them properly, you will find that they all lead you inward to the fiftieth inner gate, that of *binah*. She is the place within you that has been kept so hidden and protected that She has never been broken. Therefore She can be the beginning point of your healing, one that is nothing other than a new birth.

It is no accident, for the Zohar, that the two words *yam* and *mi*, "Sea" and "Who?" are composed of the same two Hebrew letters. *Take your most broken self, turn it around, view it from a different perspective, and it will become the Source of your healing.*

The later Kabbalists were fond of depicting their symbolic universe in the figure of a primal human form, called *Adam Kadmon*, "the primal human." Yes, they said, the lower worlds are a broken place. But the breakage only goes as far as the navel, they insisted. Above that, the divine world remains unbroken. Yours too, since you are made in the divine image. Finding *binah*, Inner Mind and Inner Mother, is what it's all about.

Mashber as "crisis" is an innovation of modern Hebrew. Eliezer Ben Yehudah's dictionary refers to it as something that had appeared "in recent times," meaning that it was not his invention. But the word does exist in a few biblical examples with the meaning of "birthing stone." It seems to have been the place where the opening or "breaking" of the womb was to take place. But it may also refer to the breaking open of the womb itself. Speaking metaphorically of Israel's situation in the face of its Assyrian enemies, King Hezekiah cries out to his priest and prophet: "Children have come to the *mashber*, but there is no strength to birth them (Is. 37:3)." The verse seems to mean that the situation is desperate, that we cannot move forward. We can understand how the modern writers got "crisis" out of this. The Yiddish writer called Der Nister even wrote a famous novel titled *Di Mishpokhe Mashber*, "The Crisis Family" (but pointing toward "the family crisis"!).

As so often happens, there is wisdom to be found in the etymologies of Hebrew words. A *mashber*, crisis, like the one we're facing now, can also serve as a *mashber*, birthing-stone, for all sorts of good things—if only we find the strength to bring them forth. A birthing-stone sounds like a pretty solid object to hold onto when you're in the midst of a whirlwind. Find one—an inner place within the crisis of this storm, hold on tight, and see what comes forth. May it be born whole and healthy!

The best-known usage of *shever* in Jewish mysticism is that of the later Kabbalists, followers of R. Yitzchak Luria in the sixteenth century, who introduced the term *shevirat ha-kelim*, "the breaking of the vessels," into the Jewish religious vocabulary. Thanks to the writings of Gershom Scholem and his school, this term is now widely familiar to readers of Jewish literature. When God created the world, so the story goes, the pure light of divine Creation was sent forth into the empty space that had been set aside as the place where the non-God might exist. The contrast between the divine and the non-divine, or the light of God's rays and the darkness of the void, was so great, however, that the vessels containing the light split apart and shattered. Bits of light and shards of broken vessels were scattered throughout cosmic space, becoming *nitsotsot*, sparks of divinity, and *kelipot*, shards or husks, that hide them.

This "accident of birth" in the process of Creation is presented in the most starkly dualistic terms. The *kelipot* are not just accidentally broken fragments, but active forces that seek to hide the light; the word *kelipah*, in later Hebrew usage as well as in Yiddish, comes to mean "demon." The motif of broken vessels is linked, already in Luria's own teachings, with other myths pointing to the existence of primal forces of evil that preceded Creation itself. Before this world was created, according to an ancient rabbinic source, there had been prior attempts at forming worlds that did not survive. The cosmic flotsam and jetsam of these earlier emanations are in turn identified with dark hints about primordial "kings," rulers of the demonic forces of Edom, who actively oppose the emergence of the present universe. All this means, in short, that the brokenness of existence has cosmic origins. It is the way the world is, and will periodically manifest itself.

This version of the Lurianic tale, however, is lacking in a key element that was necessary to permit such a Gnostic worldview to exist within the framework of rabbinic Judaism. It contains no sense of human moral responsibility. The demonic forces, and the brokenness that comes about because of them, exist in the world from the first day of Creation. Evil is inherent to existence; humans, created on the sixth day, are its victims from the moment they appear on the scene, rather than its perpetrators.

Such a view was not one that could be permitted. The tale of the breaking of the vessels was combined, for that reason (though "reason" reflects a very different mental process than that of the emerging mythic imagination), with one of the most ancient tales carried forth by the sources of Judaism—the biblical account of the first humans' sin.

Unlike early Christianity, rabbinic Judaism is not a religion in which the need to atone for an original sin plays a critical role. The early rabbis mostly believed that the struggle with evil and temptation begins over again with each person. The battle is with one's own *yetzer hara,* an inbuilt inclination toward evil (based on Gen. 8:21), but not related to the guilt of Adam over a primal sin that afflicts all humans. Indeed, a well-known Talmudic passage seems to explicitly reject such a notion: "In the hour when the snake approached Eve, he cast a poison into her. Israel, who stood at Mount Sinai, had that poison pass out of them. The nations of the world, who did not stand at Mount Sinai, did not have that poison pass away (b. Shabbat 146a). This statement, sounding horribly racist when taken at face value, seems to be a remnant of the early Jewish/Christian polemic. If you Christians want "original sin," you can have it; that is not our problem. We were wiped clean of it by accepting the Torah. The stain of sin, the passage goes on to say, returned to Israel after they worshipped the Golden Calf. This refocuses attention on the new sin of idolatry and the struggle to overcome it, rather than harking back to the sexual guilt associated with Adam and Eve. Sexual temptation, as well as idolatry in all its many forms, remain temptations within the rabbinic value system, to be sure; but the balance between the good and evil inclinations allows each person an even chance of getting things right.

But the tale of Eden does belong to our scripture, and the faint memory of a lost paradise haunts our tradition. The rabbinic rejection, or downplaying, of original sin is reversed in the kabbalistic sources. This allows for a highly confused mingling of the notion of a primal breakage built into Creation and the assumption that the first humans bore responsibility for evil in the world and the existence of the *kelipot.* Fragments of these two very distinct visions often appear together in the same work—even in the same sentence. The sense that our pre-messianic state of being is somehow "fallen" pervades the kabbalistic mentality, and we humans somehow bear responsibility for it.

This all has a suddenly familiar ring as we listen to biomedical experts discussing the origins of our current pandemic, and perhaps others to come. The microbes were here long before us; they are as much a part of the web of life as we are, and we need to accept that reality. But the danger of such calamities increases as we so rapidly destroy the habitats of other creatures, burn down rainforests, consume wild life-forms, and cross those boundaries within which humans so long have found our place. Is the universe primordially broken, or did we humans bring this upon ourselves?

Most interesting here is the Hasidic response to this prior and well-established kabbalistic conversation. Hasidism, we should remember, began as a popular religious revival movement at the end of the eighteenth century. That was the very era when the elaborate intellectual constructions of Kabbalah were beginning to collapse, partly due to outside pressures, but mostly from within. The Hasidic masters took the parts of kabbalistic language that they found useful to their revival, but left much behind. In this case, they chose the *nitsotsot*, the sparks, but not the *shevirah*, the breakage, the account of how those sparks came to be. Reading many a Hasidic source (and I beg the scholars' forgiveness for oversimplification), we find that the sparks of light were intentionally planted throughout the universe so that we might discover them, and by our joyous service reunite them with their Source. There is no essential brokenness about this world, neither that of a fault in Creation nor that of primal human sin. We see those only because of the blurriness of our vision, caused by our own sins, mainly those of chasing after our own desires and abandoning the singular quest for light. When we refocus both eyes and heart (see Num.16, the final section of the *shema*), we see before us only bits of light, waiting to be uplifted. The entire Torah is given to us as a set of tools for that work of refocusing. The *mitzvot* serve as both opportunities and paradigms for the universal human task of uplifting and transforming the world in which we live. Even this terrible hour, like many that have come before it, offers us endless opportunities to do so.

Torah in a Time of Plague

Jewish Community and Practice Under Duress

Collective Tragedy and the Jewish Politics of Mourning

Sara Labaton

Introduction

The Covid-19 pandemic has thrust people worldwide into states of loss: economic and material loss, the loss of physical and emotional well-being, the loss of routine and community, and, most profoundly, the loss of human life.[1] In the face of death, rites of personal mourning provide a structure and script for mourners to navigate their immediate grief. As the daily death tolls mount, though, it is less clear how or why a society should publicly and collectively mourn mass loss. There are certainly precedents in both American and Jewish history for collective mourning, in which a community or nation undertakes mourning for a group of people lost to tragedy. Frequently, those lost are strangers to the mourners.

Grief for strangers, however, is not intuitive, grief for a magnitude of strangers less so, and collective ritual action is difficult to orchestrate. A mass tragedy whose victims are unknown to us or whose numbers are vast does not elicit the same clear ritual avenues as personal bereavement. In contrast to personal mourning, rituals of public mourning risk appearing performative and inauthentic.

What is the purpose and meaning of public and collective mourning? What are the rituals and mechanisms that help realize these aims? The argument I propose here is that collective mourning is not meant to achieve emotional catharsis or express grief as with individual loss, but rather, is meant to realize a political opportunity. Collective mourning surfaces questions about a tragedy's roots and forces a process of social and political reckoning, which can, in turn, provoke both responses and interventions.

Jewish precedents help to illuminate political aspects of collective mourning. My focus will be on the narratives and rituals associated with

[1] I would like to thank Dan Friedman, Talia Graff, and Emily Labaton for their insightful comments on this piece, and Elisheva Urbas for her invaluable wisdom and support during the writing process.

two periods of collective mourning marked on the Jewish calendar: First, the summer mourning period for the destruction of the Temple around Tisha b'Av; and second, the seven-week period of the Omer. As we shall see, both are political in that they interrogate the underlying causes of the tragedy and seek to effect systemic change in response.

This formulation has its basis in the work of Judith Butler. In applying her prior thinking around vulnerability and mourning to Covid-19, Butler argues that collective mourning carries social, ethical, and political functions:

> A purely private form of mourning is possible but cannot assuage the cry that wants the world to bear witness to the loss. And with public losses of this magnitude and quick succession, there are political questions that are linked with the demand for public mourning: Why were health facilities so badly underfunded and unprepared? Why did the president disband the committee tasked with preparations of pandemics of this kind? Why are there not enough beds or ventilators? Why are Black people, incarcerated people and migrants more at risk of dying than those who have been afforded decent health care for years? All these lost lives are grievable, which means that they are lives worthy of acknowledgement, equal in value to every other life, a value that cannot be calculated.[2]

While the pandemic demonstrates global interconnectedness and shared vulnerability, it also exposes the unequal distribution of vulnerability. Public mourning drives structural change if it includes grief for all the lives lost and if it demands a reckoning for why some lives are more vulnerable and marked as less human than others.

In her work responding to 9/11 and the War on Terror, Butler insists that grief and mourning highlight human relationality and interdependence. When we experience loss, we lose parts of ourselves and undergo

---

[2] George Yancy, "Judith Butler: Mourning is a Political Act Amid the Pandemic and Its Disparities," Truthout.org, April 30, 2020. https://truthout.org/articles/judith-butler-mourning-is-a-political-act-amid-the-pandemic-and-its-disparities/ (last accessed September 24, 2020).

transformations or "dispossessions" precisely because these ties are constitutive of who we are. Mourning is not the resolution of grief or the restoration of an imagined reality prior to loss, but rather, the acknowledgement that the loss of another person has utterly altered the mourner herself.

Butler writes, "Many people think that grief is privatizing, that it returns us to a solitary situation and is, in that sense, depoliticizing. But I think it furnishes a sense of political community of a complex order, and it does this first of all by bringing to the fore the relationship ties that have implications for theorizing fundamental dependency and ethical obligation."[3] We clearly experience this when we lose people close to us, but Butler asks us to extend this to the experience of mass tragedy and collective loss. Maintaining grief as a political resource leads not to passivity, silence, and melancholy, but to a broader awareness of human vulnerability, common exposure to loss and violence, and the responsibility to shield others from suffering. Butler asks that her analysis of mourning be used in the service of rethinking politics and policy. An ongoing awareness of grief and vulnerability functions to create "identification with suffering itself"[4] and the consequent ethic of preventing the suffering of others.

Butler's portrait of collective mourning as a political resource stands in stark contrast to the intimate, quiet experience of mourning a personal loss, even one which unfolds in a public context. In Leviticus 10, Aaron is silent after his two priestly sons die in a divine fire, in a public spectacle that should have been a joyous consecration of the Tabernacle. Aaron's silence is not addressed in the Bible (Is he enraged? Ashamed? Submissive?), but it reads as an expression of profound aloneness. His feelings are incommunicable and there is no comfort or redemption to be found in community. However, for the Israelites silence is not tolerable and they erupt in public grief. In interrogating the meaning and message of a tragedy, collective mourning cannot allow for silence as it seeks to translate grief into action and transformation. Uncovering the systemic causes of a tragedy and weighing the correct response demand speech.[5]

---

[3] Judith Butler, *Precarious Life: The Powers of Mourning and Violence* (New York: Verso, 2004), 22.

[4] Butler, *Precarious Life*, 30.

[5] While some scholars view stunned (or, alternatively, determined) silence as the response to both the destruction of the Second Temple and the Holocaust, Jonathan Klawans uncovers the roots of that approach and compellingly argues against it. See Jonathan Klawans, "Jose-

Destruction of the Temple

Jewish mourning for Jerusalem and the Temple is communal, public, and historical. While Tisha b'Av, the fast day commemorating the two destructions of the Jerusalem Temple, serves as a proxy for mourning numerous Jewish tragedies, the primary events it recalls are embedded in a distant past. Consequently, a compound challenge of distance, magnitude, and anonymity emerges in making these mourning rituals evocative and resonant.

Rabbinic narratives written generations after the events of 70 C.E. express motives for collective mourning, namely, uncovering the underlying causes of destruction, revealing its urgent messages, and ensuring that patterns of destructive behavior do not recur. The rabbis ask repeatedly why the Temple and Jerusalem were destroyed and provide reasoning that fits within a biblical paradigm, "The destruction was a predicted, precedented, divinely orchestrated punishment for the people's transgressions."[6]

Some rabbinic texts root the destruction in a range of discrete transgressions.[7] Other reasons are couched in narratives, snapshots of morally empty and toxic lives preceding the period of the destruction as imagined by later rabbis. Texts describing the situation that preceded—and caused—the destruction are traditionally evoked during the period of Tisha b'Av, thereby embedding the pedagogic message of the destruction into the ritualized mourning for the destruction.[8] These texts function as calls for social and ethical change, insisting that later Jews absorb that lesson from the tragedy.

While a commitment to theodicy certainly runs through rabbinic reflections on the destruction, some narratives also suggest a type of human and natural causality alongside divine wrath and punishment. The famous story that unspools from the line "Jerusalem was destroyed because of

---

phus, the Rabbis, and Responses to Catastrophe Ancient and Modern." *The Jewish Quarterly Review* 100 no. 2 (Spring 2010): 278-289.

[6] Klawans, "Catastrophes," 308.

[7] Shaye J. D. Cohen, "The Destruction: From Scripture to Midrash." *Prooftexts* 2 no. 1 (1982): 25-29.

[8] During this period, an emphasis on recollection along with the injunction against typical forms of Torah study (Babylonian Talmud Ta'anit 30a) lead to a curriculum of study centering on these types of texts.

Kamtza and Bar Kamtza" (b. Gittin 55b) reads like a game of dominoes, only with stakes that get progressively higher as human behavior becomes increasingly toxic.[9] As Jeffrey Rubenstein points out, the literary structure "shifts the narrative tension from what will happen (since this is known) to how and why it happened... Crucial is the lesson that the story teaches—how and why the destruction came about, hence how to avoid such tragedies in the future."[10] Here, a personal fight,[11] public shaming, and an absence of leadership almost inevitably pave the way for civil strife, national breakdown, and even more egregious errors of leadership.

Another story, found a few pages later in the Talmud (b. Gittin 58a), uses the intersection of two relationships involving three people as a synecdoche for broader corrosion and dysfunction:

> There was **an incident involving a certain man who set his eyes on his master's wife, and he was a carpenter's apprentice.**

---

[9] In this story, an anonymous character organizes a feast and sends a servant to bring his friend Kamtza. The servant accidentally brings his enemy Bar Kamtza instead. When the host sees Bar Kamtza sitting at the feast, he orders him to leave and refuses to yield even after the latter begs and offers to pay for the entire feast. The dispute culminates with the host physically escorting Bar Kamtza out, at which point the latter decides to inform on the Sages to the king, because they sat and passively watched his humiliation without interceding. Bar Kamtza tells the emperor that the Jews have rebelled and suggests that he send a sacrifice to be brought in honor of the government as proof. The emperor proceeds to send a calf, upon which Bar Kamtza inflicts a minor blemish when bringing it to the Temple. The priests do not want to sacrifice the animal; however, they are caught in a quandary because the blemish is not one that Gentile authorities would consider invalidating. The Sages opine that the priests should sacrifice it anyway to maintain the peace, while Rabbi Zekharya ben Avkolas argues in opposition, saying that people will wrongly infer that blemished animals can be sacrificed. The Sages then suggest killing Bar Kamtza to prevent him from reporting them to the emperor for their refusal to do the sacrifice. Again, Rabbi Zakharya argues that people will draw the wrong legal inference if they do that. Consequently, nothing is done, the authorities accept Bar Kamtza's slander, and the war between the Romans and Jews begins.

[10] Jeffrey Rubenstein, *Talmudic Stories: Narrative Art, Composition, and Culture.* (Baltimore: The Johns Hopkins University Press, 1999), 148.

[11] While the narrator does not disclose the original cause of the fight, it is noteworthy that 1) the names Kamtza and Bar Kamtza do not appear elsewhere in rabbinic literature and 2) that Bar Kamtza means son of Kamtza. In addition to explaining the servant's original confusion, it is possible that Kamtza and Bar Kamtza represent a father, who is friends with the host, and a son, who is an enemy. This reading of the text coincides with the general motif of social dysfunction and strife, rooting it, first and foremost, in a family.

One time his master needed to borrow some money, and his apprentice **said to him: Send your wife to me and I will lend her** the money. **He sent his wife to him,** and the apprentice **stayed with her for three days. He** then **went back to** his master **before** she did, and the master **said to him: Where is my wife whom I sent to you?** The apprentice **said to him: I sent her** back **immediately, but I heard that the youth raped her on the way.**

The master **said to** his apprentice: **What shall I do?** The apprentice **said to him: If you listen to my advice, divorce her. He said to him:** But **her marriage contract is large** and I do not have the money to pay it. The apprentice **said to him: I will lend you** the money, and **you will give her the marriage contract.** The master **arose and divorced her,** and the apprentice **went and married her.**

When the time came that the debt was due, **and the master did not have** the means with which **to repay it,** the apprentice **said to** his master: **Come and work off your debt with me. And they,** the apprentice and his wife, **would sit and eat and drink, while he,** the woman's first husband, **would stand** over them **and serve them their drinks. And tears would drop from his eyes and fall into their cups, and at that time** the **sentence** of the destruction **was sealed.**[12]

Like the Kamtza and Bar Kamtza story, it is a human concatenation of events that leads to the final tableau of personal defeat and destruction, a life turned devastatingly upside down. In addition to exemplifying the degree of deceit and cruelty in Judean society, the story reads as a metaphor where corruption at home and work expresses national disintegration and civil strife. In this view, the portrait of a master serving his apprentice and ex-wife stands for the destruction of Judean society. Accordingly, it

---

[12] Gittin 58a, The William Davidson digital edition of the Koren Noé Talmud, Available at: <https://www.sefaria.org/Gittin.58a.21?lang=bi&with=all&lang2=en > [Accessed 24 September 2020].

is the apprentice's conniving actions and lust and the master's ignorance and naivety that engender destruction. For the authors of these two narratives, interpersonal corrosion and blatant disregard for morality tears Judean society apart. Destruction at the hands of the Romans was not simply divine punishment for various sins, but the natural and inexorable result of social decay.

By spotlighting past toxicity and demanding behavioral and societal change, the rituals used for collective and public mourning for the Temple reflect their political motivations. During the period of Tisha b'Av, rituals draw directly on the model of personal mourning. Rituals for mourning a personal loss provide structure for both spontaneous despair and for gradual, intentional reentry into community. In the words of Gordon Tucker, "Humans don't need a 'start button' for mourning. That happens naturally and automatically. What we may need is both the permission and the method for emerging from the state of grief."[13] Designated stages, starting with abstinence from ritual obligations (aninut) and including the seven-day period of sitting on the floor with torn clothes (shiva), the recitation of Kaddish, and the month-long avoidance of activities like haircuts and public joy (sheloshim), ultimately enable the mourner to return to a semblance of their past life as the intensity of the grief recedes.

In the context of collective mourning, however, Jewish tradition acknowledges the innate artifice of mourning an ancient tragedy and therefore reverses the order of the ritual stages of mourning. On the day of Tisha b'Av itself, Jews echo the shiva custom of sitting low by sitting on the floor. In the three weeks, nine days, and week leading up to this day, the pathos of grief and loss are ritually crafted through restrictions on public celebrations and haircuts (recalling the sheloshim) and by liturgical interventions to evoke memory. As Joseph Soloveitchik writes, the aspiration of "reexperience," by which a ritual event "shifts the past into the present,"[14] requires careful cultivation and staging. The norms are shaped by the realization that "However alive the experience of hurban (destruction) might be, it is nurtured by human reflection and meditation.

---

[13] Gordon Tucker, email to author, May 2020.

[14] Joseph B. Soloveitchik, *Out of the Whirlwind: Essays on Mourning, Suffering and the Human Condition*, eds. David Shatz, Joel B. Wolowelsky, and Reuven Ziegler. (Brooklyn: Ktav Publishing House, 2003), 15.

It is the intellect which commands the emotions to respond to the historical memories of the community."[15] In contrast to personal mourning, public and collective rituals of mourning strategically work to build grief, culminating with the anniversary of destruction.

The rabbis deploy the modes of personal mourning to marshal the force of Tisha b'Av's grief for the sake of change. Mourning a person in the moment is more powerful than mourning a historical, anonymous collective, a defunct institution, and an abstract tragedy. As Butler writes, "Learning to mourn mass death means marking the loss of someone whose name you do not know, whose language you may not speak, who lives at an unbridgeable distance from where you live."[16] To serve as an agent of change, collective mourning must be in dialogue with personal mourning. While it may seem inauthentic or jarring to sit on the floor on Tisha b'Av as we do with a personal shiva, it is precisely the conflation of national and personal loss that gives the moment its power.

Over the past year, the intertwining of collective and personal mourning has taken numerous forms. On Memorial Day 2020, the front page of the New York Times listed the names of nearly 1,000 Covid-19 victims, representing the 100,000 individuals lost at the time.[17] Soon after, the protests over the murder of George Floyd similarly channeled collective grief through foregrounding and mourning individual losses. Mourning individual victims of police brutality inspired global rage and calls for change in a way that the persistent reality of racial injustice has not.

Jewish tradition introduces another method of mourning the Temple, which flips mourning rituals such that instead of being powerful but momentary, they are small but pervasive. In contrast to Tisha b'Av's deployment of personal grief and mourning, this model focuses on perfunctory and banal symbols. In the Babylonian Talmud (Bava Batra 60b), this tradition comes as a response to a set of extreme grief practices proposed by a group of ascetics who are abstaining from any food or drink associated

---

[15] Soloveitchik 22.

[16] George Yancy, "Judith Butler: Mourning is a Political Act Amid the Pandemic and Its Disparities," Truthout.org, April 30, 2020. https://truthout.org/articles/judith-butler-mourning-is-a-political-act-amid-the-pandemic-and-its-disparities/ (last accessed September 24, 2020).

[17] For the background to this project, see https://www.nytimes.com/2020/05/23/reader-center/coronavirus-new-york-times-front-page.html (last accessed April 14, 2021).

with rituals once conducted in the Temple. In a conversation with these ascetics, Rabbi Joshua ben Levi rhetorically challenges them to abstain from water (also linked to a Temple ritual) to show that their approach is literally unsustainable and fatal—an obsession with death and destruction would only beget more death.[18]

Rabbi Joshua offers an alternative, a way to strike a balance between the impossibility of "not mourning at all," and "mourning overmuch...which the majority cannot endure." He cites various practices that symbolically mark the destruction through almost imperceptible diminutions. When compared to the drama of Tisha b'Av, symbolic markers such as leaving a small area of a wall unplastered, smashing a glass at a wedding, or withholding a dish from a lavish meal, may appear trivial. Unlike Tisha b'Av, however, these memorial rituals are inscribed through all of life, not just bounded by a particular frame of remembrance.

We find similar models today. In a description of the Memorial to Enslaved Laborers at the University of Virginia, Holland Cotter, a New York Times critic, writes: "Power is not its language. Closure is not its goal. Active, additive remembrance is. Is this what distinguishes a memorial from a monument? A monument says: I am truth. I am history. Full stop. A memorial says, or can say: I turn grief for the past into change for the present, and I always will."[19] In Germany, the Stolpersteine (Stumbling Stones) or the memorial resembling a simple street sign that lists twelve death camps in Berlin's Wittenbergplatz serve as examples of decidedly un-monumental memorials. Like an unplastered corner of a wall, these memorials are pedestrian (in both senses of the term) and blend into the landscape, yet they serve as ongoing reminders and calls to change. In advocating for unremarkable (even inconspicuous) commemoration, Rabbi Joshua ben Levi ensures that ambient, low-grade mourning for the Temple and its attendant messages endure beyond the intensity and theater represented by Tisha b'Av. To formulate this differently: While Tisha b'Av is thick in practice but narrow in time, Rabbi Joshua ben Levi's rituals realize an opposing impulse.

---

[18] I am grateful to Yehuda Kurtzer for this reading and insight. See Erin Leib Smokler's introduction to this volume for more insight into this story.

[19] Holland Cotter, "Turning Grief for a Hidden Past Into a Healing Space." New York Times, August 16, 2020. https://www.nytimes.com/2020/08/16/arts/design/university-of-virginia-enslaved-laborers-memorial.html.

Sefirat ha-Omer

Sefirat ha-Omer, the seven-week period stretching from Passover through Shavuot, has evolved from its biblical, agricultural, and cultic roots to become an ominous season with restrictions conventionally understood as related to mourning. In contrast to mourning the Temple, the historical basis for this general pall is obscure,[20] as is the historical link between the lachrymose mood and the restrictions. Indeed, Sefirat ha-Omer practices themselves vary widely across time and place in their details. Despite its opaque origins, however, the mourning contains a call for change, albeit one that is oriented differently than the mourning for the Temple.

The restriction on marriage for the full duration of the Omer period appears to be the earliest accepted communal norm.[21] Babylonian Geonim and early Sephardic authorities understand this restriction as mourning for Rabbi Akiva's twelve thousand pairs of students, who died, according to the Babylonian Talmud (Yevamot 62b), between Passover and Shavuot.[22] The Talmud attributes their deaths to their failure to accord one another respect. While the narrative contains distinctive literary and redactorial features,[23] the overall message reflects standard rabbinic theodicy: sin yields punishment. Mourning an ancient collective tragedy due to civil strife strongly echoes the rabbinic narratives of the Temple's destruction.[24] Unlike the mourning for the Temple for which the rabbis laid out specific practices, however, rabbinic literature lists no such practices to mourn the legendary tragedy of Rabbi Akiva's students. It is only later that various customs are tied to this event.

The medieval region of Ashkenaz displays distinctive patterns when it comes to the observance of Omer practices. According to Daniel Sperber, some of these practices were shaped by the 1096 Rhineland massacres

---

[20] Lou Silberman, "The Sefirah Season: A Study in Folklore." *Hebrew Union College Annual* 22 (1949): 221-228.

[21] Simcha Emanuel, "Minhagey Avelut Biymey Sefirat ha-Omer" [Mourning Customs During Sefirat ha-Omer]. *Netuim* 2 (2016): 109.

[22] Emanuel, 137.

[23] Aaron Amit, "The Death of Rabbi Akiva's Disciples: A Literary History." *Journal of Jewish Studies* 56 no. 2 (2005): 267.

[24] Some scholars view various restrictions associated with Rabbi Akiva's students not as mourning, but as an exercise of prudence during a dangerous time. See Emanuel, 137.

perpetrated by bands of Crusaders en route to the Holy Land. The attacks on Speyer, Worms, and Mainz occurred during the Omer period and, in response, certain Ashkenaz communities shifted the span of time during which they practiced Omer mourning to better fit the actual dates of the massacres. Whereas the traditional period of mourning fell between the second day of Passover and the thirty-third day of the Omer (the eighteenth of Iyyar), Ashkenaz communities emphasized the latter part of the Omer, when the three massacres occurred, starting from the first of the month of Iyyar through Shavuot eve.

Sperber relates this approach to the Ashkenaz practice of incorporating dirges into the Sabbath prayers during the Omer period and, idiosyncratically, of reciting Av ha-Rahamim, a prayer for the martyrs of the Rhineland massacres, even on the Sabbath before Shavuot.[25] Sperber suggests that the confluence of the Omer and the massacres also explains stringencies adopted by Ashkenaz communities. Sefer Minhag Tov, an anonymous treatise from the second half of the 13th century, describes the Omer as a platform to commemorate the Rhineland massacres:

> And it is an appropriate custom to refrain from hair cutting and buying new clothes or anything new, or to enjoy baths or cut nails from after Passover until Shavuot in honor of the pure and upright righteous ones who gave themselves over in sanctification of God's name. However, on the 33rd day of the Omer, it is permitted to do all these things due to the miracle that occurred. And from the 33rd day of the Omer through Shavuot, the stringencies stand.[26]

Sperber writes:

> ...the customs of Ashkenazic Jewry reflect the tragedy of the Persecutions of 1096 (or the Rhineland Massacres). "Crime follows crime," (lit. "Blood touches blood" see Hosea 4:2) and

---

[25] Daniel Sperber, "Minhagey Avelut be-Tequfat Sefirat ha-Omer [Mourning Customs During the Period of Sefirat ha-Omer]." *Minhagey Yisrael: Meqorot ve-Toladot* [Customs of Israel: Sources and Development] vol. 1. (Jerusalem: Mossad ha-Rav Kook, 1989), 105.
[26] Sperber, 107.

the blood of Rabbi Akiva's students flows into the seething and boiling blood of the martyrs of Ashkenaz who were killed sanctifying the Divine Name.[27]

The collective mourning for the Rhineland victims conveys a different message than the mourning linked to Rabbi Akiva's students. Using the Omer as a site for mourning later tragedies not only ensures that later losses are commemorated, but also supplies a pre-existing platform to surface other messages and call for different types of change. If mourning Rabbi Akiva's students is a call to ethical and social reform, the literature written soon after the Crusader massacres suggest two other motives for calendrically modifying and strengthening the traditional Omer mourning.

First, for Ashkenaz Jews living in the wake of the Crusades, the mourning practices of the Omer served as a way of bringing the radical, previously marginal behavior of the martyrs into the mainstream. The unprecedented feature of the Rhineland massacres was not self-sacrifice or martyrdom, but the slaughter of family members—including children—undertaken by Jews in certain communities to prevent their forced conversion. Even as the memory of these extreme expressions of martyrdom was suppressed, the attacks on the Rhineland Jews and their response elevated the status of martyrdom within the region overall.[28]

In legal, liturgical, and homiletic contexts, Ashkenaz authorities insisted upon the submission to death to avoid forced conversion. Mapping the mourning of these martyrs onto the pre-existing mourning period of the Omer canonized these specific deaths, and relatedly, changed the criteria for what was considered normative and even heroic. The Omer mourning for these martyrs was a way of changing the dominant mentality about the relevant question of when to sacrifice one's life for a religious cause.

More significantly, the Jews who were killed and martyred were considered pure and blameless, in contrast to the culpability of Rabbi Akiva's students. The Hebrew chronicles written after the events of 1096 make it clear that conventional theodicy does not work in this context. On the

---

[27] Sperber, 111.

[28] Robert Chazan, *European Jewry and the First Crusade*. (Berkeley: University of California Press, 1996), 145.

contrary, the chroniclers stress that the martyrs were greater than even Abraham, the hero of the Binding of Isaac. God, therefore, is indebted to the Jewish people, rather than the other way around. David Nirenberg claims that memorialization of the martyrs was a means to "remind God of the devotion of His people, to ensure that their payments of the ancient debts were duly noted, and even to prod God into a recollection of His covenant."[29] Anxiety around divine memory and redemption not only generated liturgy and chronicles intended to prod God, but it also, less overtly, changed the mourning practices of the Omer. Amplifying the rites associated with the Omer was a way of bringing the sacrifices of the Rhineland communities to the fore of the divine consciousness. The mourning, therefore, was not aimed at realizing internal social change, but was directed externally, at God and at the possibility of divine redemption.

Simcha Emanuel notes that the evidence linking the massacres of 1096 to the more severe Omer practices is sparse[30] and, rather, sees Ashkenaz practice take a sharp turn after the Black Death. Before the onset of the plague, major Ashkenaz authorities either ignored the Omer mourning described by the Sefer Minhag Tov or limited it to the prohibition on marriage. Following the mid-14th century, however, they expanded it to include injunctions against haircutting, nail-cutting, buying new clothing, and listening to music. In doing so, they transformed the period into one that aligns with the mourning mandated in remembrance of the Temple— and went even further, introducing restrictions once limited to mourning a family member. Emanuel attributes this to the trauma of the plague and the persecutions against the Jews that resulted in its wake. One could easily imagine that this mourning was a form of penitential prayer, intended to halt both the plague and the persecutions.

Whether Sperber or Emanuel is correct about the history of Ashkenaz customs, both scholars share an understanding of the Omer as a tool to navigate certain contemporary experiences, a template on which to map other tragedies and mourning.[31] What was relevant to Jews in Ashkenaz

---

[29] David Nirenberg, "The Rhineland Massacres of Jews in the First Crusade: Memories Medieval and Modern." In *Medieval Concepts of the Past: Ritual, Memory Historiography*, ed. Gerd Althoff, Johannes Fried, and Patrick Geary. (Cambridge: Cambridge University Press, 2002), 293.

[30] Emanuel, 116.

[31] This is, of course, not unique to the Omer. We see the same phenomenon of deploying

communities was not relevant to Jews in other regions, which resulted in severe restrictions precisely because the mourning was personal and intimate. Sperber's theory especially lays bare the different and sometimes conflicting politics and narratives to emerge from collective mourning: Are people (like Rabbi Akiva's students) at fault or is God guilty of wreaking havoc on worthy Jews? Collective mourning can serve to make meaning from tragedy, but the contours and content of that meaning change depending on the mourner and who (or what) they are mourning. Political ends differ and are often at odds, with targets as disparate as Jewish ethical behavior and divine guilt.

The use of collective mourning to force change—whether ideological in the case of making martyrdom normative or theological in either drawing God's attention to the monumental Rhineland sacrifices or pleading for a cessation to the suffering of the Black Plague—works because it is in conversation with a prior tradition and model of mourning. Apart from Holocaust Remembrance Day and Israel's Memorial Day, the Jewish calendar does not add periods of mourning. Rather, it chooses which past tragedy provides an effective frame and layers tragedies one on top of the other to mourn them simultaneously.

Conclusion

One often hears the trope of "mourning well" applied to those living in states of grief, since mourning is understood as a necessary stage for moving forward. For a society, public and collective mourning is no less of a priority because it is a means of marshalling the emotional language of grief in the service of systemic, structural, and political change. A lack of mourning reflects a lack of reckoning, without which it is impossible to re-build. In living through the pandemic and envisioning our collective response to Covid-19, Jews will be able to draw upon different models for mourning this mass tragedy. What is clear is that we must relate to it as mourners if we hope to correct the flaws in our societies that led to such massive and unequal suffering.

The Babylonian Talmud (Moed Kattan 26a) teaches that when it comes

---

pre-existing, traditional mourning for contemporary tragedies with the Ninth of Av. This is the source of some of the controversies about Holocaust Memorial Day.

to garments that were torn due to mourning, one may hem, gather, or fix them with loose and imprecise stitches, but it is prohibited to mend them fully or meticulously.[32] Maintaining an awareness of grief even after the immediate trauma subsides is a necessary form of remembrance. When it comes to collective mourning, the "torn garments" must remain in our consciousness if we are to do the necessary work of healing and rebuilding our societies.

---

[32] I thank Rabbi Neil Zuckerman for pointing me to this reference.

"A People's Multitude is a King's Splendor":
Communal Practices beyond Prayer

Ayelet Hoffmann Libson

For many people, one of the most difficult aspects of living through the age of Covid-19 is the lack of community. When fear, grief, anxiety, and loneliness abound, the Jewish response is usually to gather. Whether by bringing food to a house of mourning or by joining in prayer, Jews come together to confront adversity.

The mishnah in Tractate Ta'anit prescribes the response to various communal calamities with fasting and prayer. The most common and severe catastrophe discussed in the tractate is drought, which is met with a series of fasts over several weeks and months. According to the mishnah, as the fasts progress, prayer becomes increasingly collective. At first only select individuals fast for three fasts.[1] If rain still does not fall, the leaders decree upon the community a series of thirteen fasts, divided into three sets of increasing severity. Finally, if an extremely severe drought persists, the individuals return to fasting on their own. While at first the severity of the calamity is matched by the increased participation of the community, the most extreme response, reserved for individuals, symbolizes the breakdown of society wrought by natural disaster (m. Ta'anit 1:4-6).

The Mishnah makes it clear that shared fasts are not simply a synchronization of multiple individual fasts; rather, they are categorically different:

> What is the order [of service] for fast days? They take the ark out to the town street, and they put ashes on the head of the Nasi (Patriarch) and on the head of the head of the court. And each and every one puts [ashes] on his own head. The elder among them says before them words of admonition... (m.

---

[1] b. Ta'anit 10b suggests that these individuals are chosen based on their expertise in Torah and their ability to hear questions of Jewish law. By contrast, the Jerusalem Talmud (1:4, 64b) views the "individuals" as those known for their moral virtues and therefore expected to have their prayers answered.

Ta'anit 2:1)

The communal fast cannot take place in people's homes; it must occur in the public sphere. The visual impact is significant: The holy ark, usually ensconced within the synagogue, is taken out to the town plaza, emphasizing the significance of the moment, and perhaps making it figuratively easier to cry out to God. The leaders of the community, ordinarily those treated with the most dignity, put ashes upon their heads to demonstrate their grief and shame, and speak words of admonition to the community. This dramatic public response lends gravity to the collective prayer, underscoring the enormity of the crisis for the community. Praying together, as many of us can attest, is fundamentally different from praying alone. In his famous work, *The Elementary Forms of Religious Life*, sociologist Emile Durkheim observed that "the act of congregating is an exceptionally powerful stimulant. Once the individuals are gathered together, a sort of electricity is generated from their closeness and quickly launches them to an extraordinary height of exaltation."[2] In praying together, suggests the Mishnah, the community is greater than the sum of its parts because of the energy generated by togetherness, resulting in prayer of a different nature than that of an individual.

The power of communal prayer is discussed at various points in the Babylonian Talmud. In Tractate Yevamot 49b the rabbis distinguish between individual prayer, which is heard by God only at specific times of the year, and communal prayer, which is heard at any time, reflecting God's greater attunement to the cries of the community. Tractate Berakhot offers an extended discussion of the significance of communal prayer in several passages. In one of them we find a sequence of homilies praising communal prayer:

> It was taught that Abba Binyamin said: One's prayer is only heard in a synagogue, as it is stated, "to listen to the song and the prayer" (I Kings 8:28). In a place of song, there prayer should be.

---

[2] Emile Durkheim, *The Elementary Forms of Religious Life*. Trans. K.E. Fields (New York: Free Press, 1995/1915), 217.

Ravin bar Rav Adda said that Rabbi Yitzhak said: From where is it derived that the Holy and Blessed One is found in a synagogue? As it is stated: "God stands in the congregation of God" (Ps. 82:1). And from where is it derived that ten people who pray, the Divine Presence is with them? As it is stated: "God stands in the congregation of God." (b. Berakhot 6a)

The passage begins by maintaining that prayer is only truly heard in a synagogue, a place of communal prayer (*beit knesset*). Moreover, the second paragraph grounds the familiar idea that communal prayer is understood to consist of a minimal quorum of ten people. When ten people come together in prayer, the divine presence is found in their midst. As this generally occurs in a synagogue, that is the best place to pray.

This ideal of communal prayer has had lasting power in sustaining Jewish communities and synagogues throughout history and across the globe. Yet the Covid-19 pandemic has cast a shadow over communal prayer the world over. Some Jewish communities have continued to hold shared prayers, often at their own peril (and at great risk to others). Most praying Jews, however, have made drastic changes to their prayer routines and other ritual practices. Many have found themselves unmoored from their Jewish communities as they fled crowded urban centers for the safety of country living. Others continue to reside in their homes, but severely limit social encounters, deeming synagogue attendance unsafe. The yearning for communal prayer continues, though, as countless people have taken to technology to create virtual prayer gatherings, which have in turn spawned a host of legal questions regarding Zoom *minyans*, Zoom *seders*, Zoom *megillah* readings, Zoom weddings, and more.[3]

The desire to continue praying with a quorum of other people is certainly understandable and even laudable, particularly in light of the sources we saw advocating communal prayer to avert crisis. Nonetheless, many of us experience virtual prayer as a feeble shadow of in-person communal prayer. It is difficult to make eye-contact; singing together is impossible;

---

[3] For a survey of Orthodox responses to these questions, see Michael Broyde, "An Introduction to Pandemic Jewish Law," Tablet Magazine, April 24th, 2020. For the Conservative movement's response, see R. David Golinkin's responsa at https://schechter.edu/jewish-responses-corona-pandemic/.

and one misses the small yet pervasive gestures—the rustling of pages, the shuffling of feet, the creaking of pews. Even more than words, the choreography and cadence of prayer are crucial to creating a sense of shared purpose.

Fortunately, community is not forged by prayer alone. While rabbinic sources insist on the primacy of communal prayer, they also develop other paradigms of communal engagement that may serve to fill the void of communal prayer during the time of a plague that keeps us physically apart.

A Community of Torah Study

The first such paradigm is based on foregrounding the value of Torah study. The Mishnah teaches that the divine presence rests not only upon a community of people praying together, as we saw above, but also upon those who study Torah together:

> Rabbi Halafta b. Dosa of Kfar Hananiah says: Ten who sit together and occupy themselves with the Torah, the divine presence dwells among them, as it says: "God stands in the godly congregation" (Ps. 82:1). How do we know [that the same is true] even of five? As it says, "His band is founded upon the earth" (Amos 9:6). How do we know that even three? As it says, "In the midst of judges, God judges" (Ps. 82:1). How do we know that even two? As it says, "Then those who revere the Lord spoke to each other, and the Lord paid attention and heard" (Mal. 3:16). How do we know that even one? As it says, "In every place where I have my Name mentioned, I will come to you and bless you" (Ex. 20:20). (m. Avot 3:6)

R. Halafta's phrasing suggests that the ideal quorum of ten required for God's dwelling among people is the same whether they are engaged in study or in prayer. Yet the passage continues by gradually limiting the number of people engaged in Torah study needed to draw God into the world, until stating that even one Torah learner is enough to draw down divine blessings.

This teaching offers an alternative to our fixed ideas about praying in a *minyan* (quorum) as the pathway to communal engagement. Rather than trying to recreate our collective prayer lives through a virtual medium, the coronavirus pandemic is an opportunity to consider other approaches which might be more compatible with virtual media. When communal prayer is not possible, we can afford to free ourselves from the attempt to simply recreate communal prayer by virtual means, and instead embrace other paths to bringing godliness into our lives.

Indeed, whereas the idea of virtual prayer is a modern innovation, virtual Torah study has long precedent within Jewish tradition. The Talmud, the core text studied by generations of Jews, is inherently dialogical, a record of transhistorical conversations among scholars from different time periods and locations. The Talmud is full of debates that portray a fourth-century Babylonian sage such as Rava critiquing a first-century sage from the land of Israel, such as Hillel. The debate frequently continues with the rabbis of the Talmud offering a response to Rava's critique on Hillel's behalf. That conversation was then continued past the conclusion of the Talmud by the medieval and early modern commentators, and even into our own day. This kind of transhistorical dialogue suggests that the overarching value of Torah study can serve as a platform for bringing together students from different geographical communities as well.

The dialogical nature of Torah study has also allowed for Jews of many backgrounds—Jews who cannot pray together due to ideological differences—to learn together and from each other. As Devora Steinmetz writes, "For people who study Talmud regularly, the stories and figures of rabbinic tradition construct a universe of shared memory and meaning, a world of experience in which we participate."[4] Nowhere is this more obvious than within the circle of those who study *daf yomi*, a daily folio of Talmud, a practice initiated by R. Meir Shapiro in Poland in 1923. Today, tens of thousands of Jews study the *daf*, from ultra-Orthodox enclaves in Brooklyn and Lakewood to secular study groups in Tel Aviv and San Francisco. Despite their differences, many of these students and teachers view themselves as part of a vast virtual community of study.[5]

---

[4] Devora Steinmetz, "Talmud Study as a Religious Practice," in Paul Socken, ed., *Why Study Talmud in the Twenty First Century? The Relevance of the Ancient Jewish Text to our World* (Lexington Books, 2009), 51.

[5] For more on the study of daf yomi, see the essays by Ilana Kurshan and Ethan Leib in this volume.

The texts and practices of Torah, then, lend themselves to shared study, whether in the traditional paired format (*havruta*) or in a study group. During a pandemic, studying together by virtual means has not only social value, such as checking in on community members to make sure that they are well. Shared Torah study also affords a way to engage in meaningful content that transcends our mundane concerns and elevates life into the spiritual realm. Rabbinic tradition understands Torah to be the primary revelation of God's essence, and as such, learning Torah is a process of drawing God into the world. In sum, one path to creating meaningful community in a virtual age is a renewed commitment to the ancient practice of deep Torah study—not only as an intellectual pursuit, but as a communal devotional practice.

Shared Performance of Commandments

Another paradigm proposed by rabbinic literature for drawing a community together is the shared performance of commandments. The significance of joining together is expressed in several different ways, united under the rubric of a verse from Proverbs, "a people's multitude is a king's splendor; but without a nation a ruler is ruined" (Prov. 14:28).

Early rabbinic sources use this verse to mandate that wherever possible, one commandment should be divided amongst as many people as possible. For instance, Sifra, an early midrash on Leviticus, comments on a verse commanding each person to bring his or her offerings "to Aaron's sons, the priests" (Lev. 2:2), and explains that the verse requires a person to bring an offering not to one priest but to "the priests" as a whole, so that many priests may participate in the commandments. The Sifra supports this position with the verse "a people's multitude is a king's splendor" (Sifra, *dibura de-nedavah, par.* 9:10). In his commentary on the Sifra, R. Abraham ben David of Posquières (known by the Hebrew acronym *Raavad*) explains that each priest takes on one element: measuring the grain offering, pouring the oil, mixing, giving incense, etc. By engaging in one element of the sacrificial process, explains the *Raavad*, the priests will all come to be more engaged in and appreciative of the commandment.

The same idea is found in several passages in the Babylonian Talmud. Tractate Sukkah 52b, for instance, tells of an extraordinarily strong priest, known as the son of Marta, daughter of Baithos, who would take hold of two thighs of a bull so massive that it was purchased for a thousand coins, and walk up the ramp to the altar in the Temple without hurrying, but rather taking small steps, walking "heel to toe." His colleagues, the other priests, however impressed they were by his physical prowess, refused to let him show off, and demanded that he include as many priests as possible in the Temple service, allowing them to share the burden of carrying the sacrifice, and invoking the principle that "a people's multitude is a king's splendor."

Along similar lines, Mishnah Pesahim 5:6 teaches that after slaughtering an animal, the slaughterer would pass the bowl of blood to another priest. The Talmud (b. Pesahim 64b) expresses concern over this ruling, as passing the bowl from one priest to another might result in the blood not being "walked" to the altar, which would invalidate the sacrifice. Despite this risk, says the Talmud, this concern is overridden to underscore the principle that "a people's multitude is a king's splendor," and as many priests as possible should participate in the Temple service.

As the above sources attest, this principle originated in Temple service. But it is expanded in later sources to other communal practices. According to the medieval midrash *Leqah Tov* (*Vayera* 22), collated in 11th century Greece, during Rosh Hashanah prayers one who leads communal prayers (*shaliah tzibbur*) should not lead the blowing of the shofar; this action should be delegated to someone else. Again, the reason offered for this ruling is that "a people's multitude is a king's splendor," a particularly apt idea in the context of Rosh Hashanah and its theme of coronation. In this context, glorifying God's kingship is not an abstract idea, but rather is translated into a concrete legal ruling. God is not glorified merely by having a large nation of followers, but more particularly by having as many followers as possible participate in observing God's commandments.

In several talmudic sources, this idea is applied to commandments that can feasibly be performed by each individual, yet are more ideally fulfilled by one person *before an audience* of other obligated community members. One such commandment is the recitation of the blessing over a lit candle as part of the *havdalah* ceremony at the conclusion of Shabbat:

The Sages taught: If people were seated in the study hall and they brought a flame before them. The house of Shammai say: Each and every individual recites a blessing for himself; and the house of Hillel say: One recites a blessing on behalf of them all, as it says, "A people's multitude is a king's splendor."

Granted, the house of Hillel explains their reasoning, but what is the reason for the [opinion of the] house of Shammai? They thought [it is prohibited] because it would interrupt the study hall. (b. Berakhot 53a)

The house of Shammai maintains that each person should recite the blessing of *havdalah* individually, and the Talmud explains that their concern is the interruption of Torah learning. If everyone congregates to listen to one person recite the blessing, the flow of learning in the study hall would be compromised. That is, the house of Shammai holds that if the commandment can be performed individually, there is no value in congregating to perform it together. And if there is no value in saying the blessings performatively, in front of an audience, then how can one justify interrupting the study of Torah? The house of Hillel agrees that one can fulfill the commandment by reciting the blessing on one's own. Yet nonetheless they see great value in saying it together as a group. Moreover, the house of Hillel does not merely suggest that all those attending the study hall should stand together and each recite the blessing. Instead, one person should recite the blessing on behalf of all the observers. In contrast to the Temple-based model of dividing one commandment among many participants, the house of Hillel suggests that it is preferable that one person recite the blessing on behalf of others. Not only can one person fulfill the commandment through another person reciting the blessing, but it is in fact preferred that only one person recite the blessing, because this leads to everyone in the study hall congregating together. What at first seems like a legal quibble actually reveals a profound theological truth: Performing a commandment is certainly an act of doing God's will, yet coming *together* to perform commandments is an act of glorifying and magnifying God.

The King's Splendor

The key to understanding the value of shared performance of the commandments lies in examining the verse from Proverbs that serves as the underlying reasoning for this rabbinic concept. "A people's multitude is a king's splendor, but without a nation a ruler is ruined" (Proverbs 14:28). Whereas the metaphor of God as king and Israel as God's nation is a ubiquitous one in biblical literature, generally this metaphor conveys the people's dependence upon God.[6] By contrast, the focus of the verse in Proverbs is on God's dependence on God's people. While to his subjects, a king may seem mighty and distant, this verse reveals that the king is in profound need of his people. In fact, he may even need them more than they need him! Without his followers, the king has nothing: not power, not riches, not honor, nor fame.

The radical idea of a king's dependence upon his followers is developed in *Sifre Zuta*, an early rabbinic commentary on the book of Numbers. The midrash comments on the dialogue between Moses and his father-in-law, Jethro, in which Moses pleads with Jethro, "please do not leave us, for you know where we should camp in the wilderness and can serve as our eyes" (Num. 10:31). Focusing on the enigmatic phrase "serve as our eyes," the midrash subverts the plain meaning of the verse and its focus on the needs of the children of Israel in the desert, and instead reads this phrase to refer to "the eyes of all humankind" (*kol ba'ei olam*). The midrash maintains that should Jethro depart, all the people of the world will employ an *a fortiori* argument. If even Moses' father-in-law was not welcome amongst the children of Israel, all the more so would other proselytes be rejected. According to this logic, Moses chides Jethro by arguing:

> You will be found to be distancing proselytes from joining us and from enhancing divine honor (*kevodo shel makom*), to fulfill what is written "a people's multitude is a king's splendor." (Sifre Zuta 10:31)

---

[6] On the metaphor of divine kingship, see Yochanan Muffs, *The Personhood of God: Biblical Theology, Human Faith and the Divine Image* (Woodstock, VT: Jewish Lights, 2005), 78-81.

Moses' rebuke assumes that a king is defined by his followers' approval and desire to be part of his nation. The best indicator of approval for a king is outsiders' wishes to join his kingdom. If Jethro leaves the children of Israel, he will unintentionally discourage others from joining Israel—thereby decreasing God's splendor, argues Moses. The underlying assumption of this argument is that God needs followers, and the more followers, the better.

A later midrash, however, suggests that God does not merely want many followers, but rather desires a relationship particularly with Israel:

> "A people's multitude is a king's splendor, but without a nation the ruler is ruined." R. Hama bar Hanina said: Come and see the praise and greatness of the Holy and Blessed One, that although he has a thousand thousands of thousands and hundreds of thousands of groups of angels to serve and praise Him, He does not want their praise, but rather the praise of Israel, as it says, "A people's multitude is a king's splendor..." (Midrash *Mishlei* 14:28)

This homily emphasizes the exclusive relationship between God and God's people. According to R. Hama b. Hanina, it is not so much that God wants to be praised in general, but rather that God wants to be praised by *Israel*. Indeed, the midrash subsequently cites another verse—"The people I formed for Myself, that they might declare my praise" (Isa. 43:21)—and interprets it to mean that the sole reason for Israel's creation is to praise God: "in order that they might declare my praise in the world" (ibid.).

Yet the rabbis did not leave this idea in the abstract; instead, they developed it concretely in legal terms, as we saw above. God is praised by observing God's commandments, and by doing so in community. Commandments performed publicly are to be divided into parts so as to include as many people as possible. And commandments that cannot be divided should be performed by one person in front of the community, so that all may congregate and serve as an audience for the blessings recited over the commandments.

In his book *Community*, Peter Block suggests that we can always form new ways of creating community. "The future is created one room at a time, one gathering at a time," he writes. "Each gathering needs to become an example of the future we want to create."[7] Block imagined people assembling together in a physical room, but the same is true of meetings in virtual space or in backyards: each gathering sets the terms for the next. When we are unable to stand in the town street and put ashes on our heads, and when we must refrain from congregating in synagogues, the principle of "a people's multitude is a king's splendor" may still abide in new and interesting ways.

Rabbinic tradition offers us a language grounded in Jewish law for looking at communal ritual in a different way. Even if we cannot fulfill the legal obligation of communal prayer by virtual means, showing up to glorify God together still holds significance as observing a Jewish duty. For those who are inspired by virtual prayer, the rabbinic principle of "a people's multitude is a king's splendor" reframes that activity in a ritually and halakhically meaningful way. And for those exasperated with trying to recreate a community of prayer in the virtual world, viewing other paradigms as equal glorification of God allows us to turn to other avenues, such as studying together or engaging in Jewish ritual, that are more amenable to virtual media. Through shared Torah study or communal performance—and maybe even through virtual prayer—we just might be able to build a sense of community, despite—or because of—the plague. One Zoom room at a time.

---

[7] Peter Block, *Community: The Structure of Belonging* (San Francisco: Berrett-Koehler Publishers, 2008), 93.

Collectivism and Individualism in the Time of Plague: How We Stand

Jon A. Levisohn

1

Writing this essay in the midst of a pandemic, it seems like a very long time since Jews gathered in synagogues in healthy numbers on a regular basis—since they stood together as they did before everything changed in March 2020. Gatherings do happen, of course. They happen online; they happen outside with distancing; they even happen in small numbers dispersed within large sanctuaries. But those gatherings are not instances of standing together in the same sense. Does this matter? Does it matter how we stand?

The reminder or remonstration, *"Da lifnei mi atah omed"* ("Know before Whom you stand") is often inscribed in a prominent location in synagogues. Each individual person who stands before that inscription—paradigmatically during the Amidah, the "standing prayer" uttered by each congregant silently to themselves—is enjoined to perform a mindful act of the imagination, to envision themselves as standing before the Divine. The formula does not emphasize God's presence ("Know that God is present") or even point to broader behavioral implications ("Always act as if God is present"), although perhaps those elements are implicit. Instead, the inscription recommends a particular stance, in the literal sense of the word.

How does one actually accomplish this? For some Jews, the biblical accounts of revelation may serve as models, since those accounts are mostly cases of individuals who experience some extraordinary circumstance. Thus, some may imagine themselves standing before a burning bush, like Moses (Exod. 3). They may imagine themselves before an elaborate technicolor vision of Divine creatures, like Ezekiel (Ezek. 1). Or perhaps they imagine themselves all alone in a cave in the wilderness, experiencing a "still small voice," like Elijah (1 Kings 19).

In the standard case, a person standing in synagogue is not standing alone but rather alongside a congregation. Prayer within Judaism is primarily communal, not individual: Most prayers are framed grammatically in the plural, and the most central prayers known as *devarim she'bi'kedushah* (loosely, "sacred utterances") are traditionally restricted to public and shared performance in the presence of a minyan, a quorum of ten. Nevertheless, while standing alongside others, each individual may stand alone, with their own innermost thoughts and emotions, before the Divine. *"Da lifnei mi atah omed"* suggests not only that they *may* do so, but that they *must* do so. "Prayer, for all its public features," Shalom Carmy writes, "is fundamentally an affair between [the individual] and God."[1]

What is the source for this common inscription? According to a story in the Talmud (b. Berakhot 28b), the students of Rabbi Eliezer approach him on his deathbed and beg him for his final teaching "in the ways of life, that we may merit life in the world to come." He offers them four directives, the last of which is that, "when you are praying, you should know before Whom you stand." For centuries, Rabbi Eliezer's directive has inspired the interior designers of synagogues.

In the text, Rabbi Eliezer's teaching is in the plural (*"de'u"* in the second person plural imperative, i.e., "you (pl.) should know," rather than *"da"* in the second person singular masculine imperative). This fits with the narrative, since he is speaking to multiple students. But for those who are familiar with the synagogue inscription, the discrepancy is notable. At some point, someone—a rabbi, a scribe, an architect or artisan—decided that, for the purposes of immortalizing Rabbi Eliezer's words on the synagogue walls, a grammatical transition was necessary. Make no mistake, that early interior designer opined; Jews in close physical proximity to other Jews in a synagogue ought nevertheless to see themselves as individuals standing before God.

2

At the beginning of the Book of Numbers, God says to Moses, "Take a census of the whole Israelite community, by their clans and ancestral

---

[1] Shalom Carmy, "Solitary prayer," First Things, August 2020. Available online: https://www.firstthings.com/article/2020/08/solitary-prayer, accessed July 14, 2020.

houses" (Num. 1:2). Why? The very first gloss in the book (on Num. 1:1) by the great 11th century exegete Rashi offers an explanation: "Because God loves them, he counts them repeatedly," and then mentions three separate instances of counting in the biblical text. Counting is an act of love.

Rashi's commentary here echoes his earlier commentary on Exodus 30:16, where he links the census there to the preceding episode of the Golden Calf and the ensuing retributive plague. Drawing on Midrash Tanhuma (Ki Tisa 9), Rashi offers a parable.[2] The Israelites are like a flock of sheep, "beloved by its master," that is likewise "struck by a plague." When it is over, the master asks the shepherd to count the remaining beloved sheep. God is the master in this parable, and Moses the shepherd.[3] Of course, the plague itself is a punishment from God. Still, God apparently feels the need to express Divine love despite—or perhaps precisely because of—the preceding destructive expression of Divine anger.

In his commentary on Numbers 1:1, Rashi does not cite the entire parable, but his language unambiguously echoes his commentary in Exodus. What is new in Numbers is the additional element of repetition. Counting as an act of love is not simply a response to loss or grief, and not simply an emotional pendulum-swing from the expression of destructive anger. It may also reveal a compulsion, the way that a collector might repeatedly revisit the items in her collection. Either way, what matters in the counting is not the outcome of the count, the arithmetic sum. A person counts and recounts not because she needs to know how many items there are, but because the process of the count serves some emotional need. So, too, the individuation of souls on the part of the Divine is an expression of love, as each person receives their own fleeting moment of attention.

In the 12th century, Rashi's grandson Rashbam rejects his interpretation. For him, the purpose of the census is straightforward. All you have to

---

[2] The version in the Tanhuma is dry and technical, without the emotion that Rashi invests in it: If a wolf were to attack a flock, the owner would direct the shepherd to count the sheep that are left to find out how many are missing. The notion that the owner loves the sheep, and grieves their loss, is entirely absent.

[3] The effectiveness of the parable is bolstered by the fact that the biblical Moses is himself a shepherd. It is also worth noting that the image of God as shepherd and the people as sheep is found elsewhere as well, without the emphasis on counting and individuation (for example, Ezekiel 34:12: "As a shepherd seeks out his flock when he is among his sheep that are separated, so will I seek out My sheep…").

do is notice the dates: The census takes place on the first day of the second month (Num. 1:1), and less than three weeks later, on the twentieth day of the second month, the Israelites break camp and embark for Canaan (Num. 10). Obviously, the purpose of the census is to prepare for the upcoming military campaign.

Rashbam's view is strengthened by the fact that the text explicitly says that the census should include all those who are *"yotz'ai tzavah"* (Num. 1:3), which we might loosely translate as "suitable to be conscripted to the army." Nehama Leibowitz adds that the exclusion of the Levites, because of their particular cultic (i.e., non-military) role, is further support for Rashbam's view—and is hard to square with Rashi's.[4] Counting is not an act of love. It is not primarily about individuation and focusing on each person. Counting has a functional purpose that is related to the collective. For Rashbam, we could say, there is particular power in standing before God en masse, shoulder to shoulder, undertaking a communal responsibility. God's counting is a prelude, or even a call, to a shared mission.

3

In the interpretive competition between these two images—the image of standing before God as an individual versus the image of standing before God as a collective—Rashbam has the stronger argument based on the immediate textual context. Based on the broader textual context, on the other hand, Rashi has a stronger argument; his explanation accounts for the larger data set of multiple countings. (Thus, it is insufficient to simply refer to Rashbam's interpretation as *peshat*, i.e., the plain sense of the text, and Rashi's as *derash*, the allusive or homiletical sense.) But regardless, on the theological question, the Jewish tradition has embraced Rashi's view. The idea of standing before God as individuals, receiving God's loving attention, is firmly entrenched.

Nowhere is this more evident than in *Unetaneh Tokef* ("Let us now recall..."), the revered High Holy Day liturgical poem or *piyyut*.[5] The

---

[4] Nehama Leibowitz, *Studies in Bamidbar (Numbers)*, translated by Aryeh Newman (Jerusalem: World Zionist Organization, 1980).

[5] In the 13th century, Rabbi Isaac ben Moses of Vienna recorded a tradition according to which the poem was composed by one Rabbi Amnon (about whom nothing is known) around the 11th century, but scholars believe that it is actually significantly older than that—prob-

central image is of each soul passing before God's judgment.

> The great shofar is sounded
> and only a still small sound is heard.
> The angels are alarmed, gripped with fear and trembling...
> The whole of mankind pass before You like a flock of sheep.
> Just as a shepherd counts his flock
> by passing them one by one under his staff,
> so do You pass and count and enumerate and inspect every
> living soul,
> and decide the fate of every creature,
> and inscribe their verdict.

The entire poem is about—and is designed to elicit—fear and awe. But as terrifying as it might be to receive God's unwavering judgmental attention, the central image undeniably evokes the loving parable that we saw in Rashi, that is, an image of each individual being counted one by one.

The piyyut even incorporates the trope of counting, which really makes no sense here. The judge who looks down at the defendant on trial is not *counting* that defendant, no matter how many defendants have come before and how many are still waiting to be tried. But as we saw in Rashi, there is a midrashic link between the counting of sheep and the counting of people, with both sides of the parable representing a loving, individuating gaze.[6] The poet does not need to specify that God loves God's creatures; the intertextualities do that work for him.

As we dig deeper, however, the story gets more complicated. *Unetaneh Tokef* itself is based on a mishnah (Tractate Rosh Hashanah 1:2) and its

---

ably from the 6th or 7th century, the classical period of piyyut in Byzantine-era Palestine. See, for example, Reuven Kimelman's article from 2011 (Kimelman, Reuven, "U-N'Taneh Tokef as a Midrashic Poem," in *The Experience of Jewish Liturgy: Studies in Dedicated to Menachem Schmelzer*, edited by Deborah Blank Reed. Leiden: Brill. 115-146), and the scholarship cited there. My operating assumption here is that Rashi, in the 11th century, knew the liturgical poem and was influenced by it, but I have not researched this further.

[6] The word "sheep" in English, like its counterpart in Hebrew, can be a collective singular noun, which can suggest that we envision the whole flock as a collective. That is why the image of the shepherd counting sheep is so significant, because it emphasizes the individuation of each sheep within the collective.

accompanying talmudic interpretation. According to the mishnah, there are four different judgement days in the year—one for produce, one for fruit, one for water, and one in which "the whole of mankind pass before Him like a flock of sheep." The last day, of course, is Rosh Hashanah.

The phrase "the whole of mankind..." is exactly the same phrase used in the poem. In other words, the piyyut quotes the mishnah. But the Hebrew term "*kivnei maron*" in the phrase, translated above as "like a flock of sheep," is actually quite obscure. Thus, the Babylonian Talmud (Rosh Hashanah 18b) presents a menu of possible translations:

> What is *kivnei maron*?
> Here [in Babylonia], they translate it as "like a flock of sheep."
> Reish Lakish says, "Like the ascent of Beit Maron."
> Rabbi Judah says in the name of Samuel, "Like
> the troops of the Davidic monarchy."

Three opinions, none of them quite convincing on philological grounds, each offering a very different image.

For the author of *Unetaneh Tokef*, the correct answer was clear. When the poet envisioned what it means to stand before God, he was captivated by the image of God as judge of each individual. Just as each individual gets their own moment of Divine attention in the process of counting, so too, but in a more terrifying way, each individual gets their own moment of Divine attention in the process of judgment.

But for Rabbi Judah in the talmudic passage just quoted, the mishnah is properly understood to declare that, on Rosh Hashanah, "all of mankind pass before God like the troops of the Davidic monarchy." The image is not one of shepherds counting their sheep one by one. Instead, the image is of a military parade, an army marching in formation, or passing, as we say, "in review." To be sure, there is an element of judgment here—but it is a judgment of the collective, not a judgment of each individual. Even if an individual soldier steps out of line, the problem with that act of noncompliance is the effect on the cadence and chemistry of the whole.[7] The

---

[7] Without diving into the history of military parades, and of precision marching in particular, my assumption is that Roman armies employed these elements (parades and marching) and thus that Jews in Roman Palestine were familiar with them.

purpose of the review is not the judgment of each individual; the purpose is a judgment of the collective.

In fact, we can say even more than this. If an individual is judged, we can assume that a positive evaluation brings credit to that individual. If a collective is judged (perhaps a dance troupe or a team in a team sport), again, the positive evaluation brings credit to the group. The curious thing about military parades is that the honor and the glory flow back to the *reviewer*, the ruler or the general to whom the troops are loyal. As we read in Proverbs 14:28, "A large number of people brings glory to a king." Even a parade celebrates not the marchers directly but the cause for which they are marching or the occasion on which they march. If this is what happens on Rosh Hashanah, then the very meaning of Rosh Hashanah has dramatically shifted—from the day of judgment to the day of royal military parades.[8]

We are still left with the puzzle about how the Mishnah could employ a term, *"kivnei maron,"* that was so unintelligible just a few generations later that it led to diametrically opposed interpretations. The answer to that puzzle becomes clear when we examine the oldest manuscripts of the Mishnah, where it becomes clear that *"kivnei maron"* is a typo.[9] The original phrase was *"kivenumeron,"* "like a *numerus*, a military regiment," as is evident below in the image from the 12th century Kaufmann Manuscript.[10]

---

[8] There are other rabbinic sources beyond m. Rosh Hashanah 1:2, of course, that do seem to present the more familiar idea of Rosh Hashanah as a day of judgment of individuals (for example, b. Rosh Hashanah 16b, which offers the image of three books that are open on Rosh Hashanah). Likewise, there are other rabbinic sources that present the idea of God's love of individuals (for example, Rabbi Akiva's teaching in m. Avot 3:14, "Beloved is the human being, who is created in the image [of God], and it is an extraordinary love that he is conscious that he is created in the image [of God]").

[9] Aharon Oppenheimer, *Between Rome and Babylon* (Tubingen: Mohr Siebeck, 2005), p. 185; J. N. Epstein, *Introduction to the Text of the Mishnah* (Hebrew) (Jerusalem: Magnes Press, 1964), p.722.

[10] The image from the manuscript makes it clear that the fourth letter (of the second word on the second line) is a vav rather than a yod, and the vocalization is "kivenumeron" rather than "kivnei maron." Images of the Kaufmann Manuscript are available online in a number of places, including at http://kaufmann.mtak.hu/index-en.html. The image for m. RH 1:2 is at http://kaufmann.mtak.hu/en/ms50/ms50-075r.htm.

מראה שהשעה כל באי העולם עוברים
לפניו כבנו מירון שנ היוצר יחד לבם

We do not possess manuscripts of the Mishnah from before the time of the Babylonian Talmud, of course, but still, we can discern a fairly straightforward and plausible sequence of events. Here is how Simchah Roth explains it:

> The original text [of the Mishnah] read that all mankind passes before Him "kivenumeron," as in a regiment... When this term was no longer understood the text was "emended" to read "kivnei maron," which yields little sense, but can be understood somehow [according to the first opinion in the Talmud] as meaning "a flock of sheep." This corrupt reading of the text gave rise to the beautiful image in the liturgical prose-poem of the high holidays, "*U-netanneh Tokef*," of God counting all human souls as a shepherd counts his flock passing them one by one under his crook.[11]

We might only add that Rabbi Judah, the third view in the Talmud, who "translated" the phrase as referring to a military parade, clearly had a tradition that coheres with the original term *kivenumeron*. Over time, however, the first view won out. What happens on Rosh Hashanah? Each individual soul is judged by God. By the time of the composition of *Un-etaneh Tokef* in the 6th or 7th century, everyone knows what Rosh Hashanah is all about—not a day of royal military parades but the day of judgement.

The story of this mishnah, then, presents us again with two possibilities for what it means to stand before the Divine—standing as an individual or standing as a collective. The reception history seems to favor the former over the latter. What began as an image of standing as a collective evolved

---

[11] Simchah Roth, Hashkafah Study Group of the Bet Midrash Virtuali of the Rabbinical Assembly in Israel, originally published on September 20, 1998. Available online at http://www.bmv.org.il/shiurim/hashkafah/special3.asp, accessed July 14, 2020.

over time to an image of standing as an individual.

Circling back to the interpretive debate about the census in Numbers 1, we might also say that Rashbam's emphasis on collective responsibility and shared mission echoes the original meaning of *kivenumeron*. When God directs Moses to count the people, Rashbam is saying, let's imagine that moment of Divine attention as being focused on the collective. On the other hand, Rashi is promoting the alternative idea. His focus on Divine love for and attention to each individual echoes the evolved meaning of Rosh Hashanah, as it appears in the first opinion in the Talmud and as it appears in *Unetaneh Tokef*—the image that won out over time—of standing before God as individuals, receiving God's loving gaze.

4

To propose that one image of standing before the Divine came to dominate the Jewish imagination is not to say that it did so exclusively. It is certainly the case, as we noted at the outset, that most of the biblical accounts of revelation are of individuals who experience some extraordinary circumstance (Moses, Elijah, Ezekiel, and others). But the central biblical account of revelation is the collective experience of the Divine at Sinai. Setting aside the complicated and contradictory choreography (in Exod. 19) of approaches to the mountain and retreats from it, ascents and descents, the picture in the text is clear: The people were present *en masse*.

In what is perhaps the most famous midrash about that collective experience, Rabbi Avdimi (in b. Shabbat 88a) employs a hyper-literal reading of the straightforward phrase "*be-tahtit ha-har*," "at the base of the mountain" (Exod. 19:17), which he intentionally misreads to mean "underneath the mountain."

> Rabbi Avdimi b. Hama b. Hasa said: [This phrase, "underneath the mountain,"] teaches that the Holy One held the mountain over them like a barrel and told them, "If you accept the Torah, then all will be good. Otherwise, this will be your grave."

Apparently, God had to threaten the people into accepting the Torah.

The midrash, however, continues with a rebuttal in the name of Rabbi Aha who, like any good legalist, knows that a coerced agreement is no agreement at all.

> Rabbi Aha b. Jacob said: This provides a powerful legal disclaimer regarding the [acceptance of the] Torah.

If we take Rabbi Avdimi's midrashic reading seriously, Rabbi Aha says, then the covenant is not actually binding on the Jewish people.[12]

Rabbi Aha's objection is straightforward and obvious, so much so that we might wonder why Rabbi Avdimi would propose to tell us the story of the mountain over the heads of the people in the first place. What lesson does he hope we will learn from this image?

Perhaps Rabbi Avdimi simply believes in a coercive God: God commands and humans must obey. Whether this is fair or just according to the legal models with which we are familiar, whether it is an attractive picture of the Divine or a repulsive one, it is unavoidably how things are. Or perhaps, slightly differently, this is how Rabbi Avdimi himself experiences the world: God acts, and humans suffer. In spinning his yarn, perhaps he simply wants to propose that we will be better off if we know this up front, rather than persisting in the fantasy of a warm and loving God.

However, there's an entirely different way of reading Rabbi Avdimi in the midrash. We have been assuming that, when God holds the mountain over the heads of the people, the mountain is a weapon. Holding up the mountain is like pointing a gun at someone's head. God had some interest in coercing the people, so God reached out, as it were, to the nearest implement at hand, which happened to be the entire mountain.

But that's an unsatisfying way to read the symbolism of the mountain. Instead, we might read more closely and notice that there is a kind of structural similarity between God's gesture and God's words: God holds up

---

[12] As the passage continues, a third sage, Rava, comes along and saves the day with a stunningly bold interpretive move, claiming that the Jews in the time of Esther "confirmed [voluntarily] that which they had already accepted [coercively]." While we don't have time to explore this move in depth, we should at least notice the way that Rava relocates the covenant from the grand moment at Sinai to an apparently inconsequential moment many years later, from a time when the Divine is dramatically visible and audible to a time when the Divine is, famously, hidden.

the mountain and then says, "If you accept the Torah..." The immediate antecedent of "the Torah" is the mountain that God, holding it over the people, is *offering* to the people. The mountain, in the gesture, is parallel to the Torah, in the words. The mountain represents the Torah. We might therefore add an interpretive interpolation: "If you accept this thing that I am offering, that I am holding out *over* you but also *to* you, this Torah which is like a mountain..."[13]

If we imagine that the mountain represents the Torah itself—if we imagine that it represents all those commitments and obligations, formal and informal, that are the very stuff of human life, as we strive to create meaning and purpose and goodness in the world, and that are called by the rabbis "the yoke of the commandments," the burden that rests on one's shoulders that, like the yoke on a beast of burden, is both a weight and a guide—then "accepting the Torah" in the midrash does not mean that God tosses the mountain to the side with a flick of the Divine hand. It is not the case that, upon getting the coerced response, God defuses the weapon of mass destruction. Instead, "accepting the Torah," accepting the "yoke of the commandments," means shouldering the burden. We might think about the classical figure of Atlas, holding up the entire world. Unlike Atlas, though, in this case the world does not rest on the shoulders of a single heroic individual. Instead, the mountain comes to rest on the shoulders of the entire nation, standing together.

What, then, is Rabbi Avdimi trying to teach us? Perhaps the point of the image is that there is much within the Divine relationship, as in the rest

---

[13] The image of the mountain suspended in the air calls to mind a parallel image: "The laws of Shabbat, festival offerings (chagigot), and misuses of sanctified property (me'ilot) are like mountains suspended by a hair, for they have few textual sources and many laws" (m. Hagigah 1:8). In both images, a mountain seems to be unnaturally suspended in mid-air; it is hard to imagine that the two images are not in dialogue. In the Hagigah image, however, there is nobody underneath the suspended mountain, so it does not pose a threat to anyone. Moreover, in the Hagigah image, while there is physical tension (the hair might snap due to the weight of the suspended mountain), there is no dramatic tension (the situation does not need to be resolved, and if the hair is strong enough, the mountain might just stay exactly where it is). Yet, on my reading of the Shabbat image, the mountain represents the Torah (which is to say, human obligations) just as the Hagigah image suggests. More generally, I am proposing that we should interpret the Shabbat image in light of the Hagigah image, de-emphasizing precisely the two distinctions of the threat and the need for resolution. Instead, like the Hagigah image, the Shabbat image too is a way of characterizing an aspect of religious experience that persists.

of human experience, that feels literally unbearable if we imagine trying to do so alone. It will destroy us. However, if we can build the bonds of solidarity between us, if we can create or recreate the commons, if we can pursue the interest of all with hope rather than pursuing our own interests in fear, then we can shoulder any burden.

Rabbi Avdimi says: Imagine a mountain hanging over a people. Now imagine that people, unified, welcoming that burden, letting it come to rest, confident that what would crush any one of them will be borne by them all. If they accept the burden under those conditions, then all will be good.

5

Religion may well be, as Alfred North Whitehead wrote, "what the individual does with his own solitariness," at least in certain respects.[14] With Rashi, we humans—especially moderns—may well gravitate to the image of God's loving gaze falling upon each of us as individuals, like sheep. "Know before Whom you stand" may well remind us to envision a personal connection to the Divine. In times of trouble or of existential loneliness, God's love may feel like—may actually *be*-our salvation.

For many of us, this emphasis on the individual accords with our own sense of what's important, ethically and spiritually. It affirms our individuality and autonomy, our sense that a full life is one that is chosen freely and with responsibility. We stand on our own two feet.

Yet in this time of plague, of separation and isolation that feels unrelenting, the limitations of this stance become more obvious and more tragic. What we want and need more than anything else is not to be seen as individuals, not to pursue our own projects, but to stand together with others even at some cost to our individuality. We want to be counted in the collective. We want to join the shared project, to be subsumed in the shared mission. We don't need to march to the beat of a different drummer; we would be happy to march in lockstep.

As in the commentary of Rashbam on Numbers 1:1, the kind of counting that counts now is not the individuation of the sheep by the loving

---

[14] Alfred North Whitehead, *Religion in the Making: Lowell Lectures* (Cambridge: Cambridge University Press, 1926).

shepherd, but preparation for a collective mission. As in the view of Rabbi Judah on the meaning of Rosh Hashanah, the evaluation that we envision is a collective one; not how well *I* did this year but how well *we* are doing, showing up *en masse*. As in the image proposed by Rabbi Avdimi, we know that the burdens we face are unbearable if we try to stand alone, but that shouldering those burdens can be the very shared purpose we seek—if we stand together.

Household and Halakha in a Time of Pandemic

Deena Aranoff

Traditional Jewish practices can turn household tasks into ceremonial ones. What we eat, how we keep time, with whom we gather—all of these elements acquire an acute ritual status when lived in a halakhic mode. The customs that have guided Jewish behavior for millennia, first attested in biblical materials and continuously generated through the interaction of tradition and circumstance, can transform the routine flow of human activity into marvelous palaces of time.[1]

How does a pandemic affect traditional religious life? On the one hand, halakhic practices can provide comfort during a time of strain. They allow one to maintain a regular, purposeful course of action even when circumstances spin into radical uncertainty. For example, the pandemic poses a unique challenge to our efforts to keep time. Time is many things, but it is most certainly the product of collective human rhythms and routines. The sudden dissolution of these routines has sent our gaze toward a crushing, unbroken temporal horizon. Sacred rituals have the potential to break up this daunting time span and to establish behavioral patterns that link us to the seasons, to sunset and nightfall, to a collective history, and to the community of people inhabiting the same sacred calendar. As Michael Fishbane wrote years ago, "The calendar is the true Jewish theology."[2] Traditional practices can draw a person into the arc of a collective history and into the more immediate web of a community. Indeed, they can provide for assembly without assembly. Keeping time with one another, it turns out, is another way to gather.

At the same time, living in a state of crisis can also erode halakhic

---

[1] This phrase is drawn from Abraham Joshua Heschel's majestic study of the Sabbath and its temporal dimensions. A. J. Heschel, *The Sabbath*, xv-xvi. In her recent scholarship, Charlotte Fonrobert has emphasized the spatial dimensions of Shabbat as it sacralizes not only time but space, including homes and neighborhoods. Charlotte Fonrobert, "Gender Politics in the Rabbinic Neighborhood: Tractate Eruvin," in Tal Ilan, Tamara Or, Dorothea M. Salzer, Christiane Steuer and Irina Wandrey, eds., *A Feminist Commentary on the Babylonian Talmud, Introduction and Studies* (Tübingen: Mohr Siebeck, 2007), 44.

[2] Michael Fishbane, *Judaism: Revelation and Traditions* (San Francisco: Harper Collins, 1987), 83.

sensibilities. The primal energies that are summoned toward halakhic practices are the very same energies that are occupied in the face of the pandemic. The work to ensure our access to food and basic supplies, to organize and clean our homes, to tend to our social and family bonds—all of these activities are impossibly weighed down by efforts to manage the conditions of the pandemic. Let us consider, for example, the cycles of Shabbat and festivals. In the best of times, these holidays usher in a frenzy of activity for Jewish households. Special foods are prepared; invitations are issued or accepted for meals and social visits. At the appropriate time, we hope to find ourselves at tables filled with family and friends where we will repeat the stories of our ancestors, sing the songs of our families, and eat the recipes that have graced our tables for generations. In all other years, these activities form a welcome disruption to the unremarkable flow of our routine lives. This year we ask: How can we adorn ourselves in the garments of tradition when our lives have been upended by the dictates of the pandemic? How can we embrace the demands of halakha when we lack our basic routines, which, it turns out, may have functioned as a necessary backdrop to these ritual alterations? Put in halakhic terms, we are living in a semi-perpetual circumstance of *pikuach nefesh* (saving a life)—a halakhic concept that suspends all other considerations in deference to the imperative to pursue life. What happens to halakhic sensibilities when we must constantly assess our ritual behaviors in light of grave dangers and risks? How do we create sacred time in an age of pandemic?

I believe we have two options before us. The first is to determine that there are simply no energies left for ceremony. All our energies are accounted for in the effort to stay healthy in the face of the virus. The second option is perhaps more life-affirming. We might consider that there is a bit of energy available—like the fabled jar of oil that lit the Temple for eight full days; energy that, if well-spent, may provide comfort and elevation in this time of uncertainty. It is this second path that I would like to explore here.

Judaism is particularly well-suited for the continuity of ritual life in the circumstances of pandemic for one specific reason: much of Jewish ritual takes place in the home. The devastation of social life wrought by the pandemic has left one institution standing: the household. No longer complemented by the robust social life of the neighborhood, park, school or *shul*, the household has become the semi-exclusive site for social life, and, by extension, Jewish life. This isolation has imposed immeasurable and painful difficulties upon many, as most households rely upon an array of complementary spaces and relationships for support. The crises of childcare, eldercare, social isolation, and economic devastation loom large. For the purposes of this essay, however, we will focus upon the heightened significance of the household as the single domain for Jewish living and the challenge and opportunity that this presents. The hardships endured during a pandemic can eat away at even the strongest religious commitments. At the same time, perhaps due to the strain endured during this time, even the smallest ritual action can suffuse the isolated household with purpose and vitality.

Household and Halakha: A New Genealogy

The centrality of the household in Jewish life is well known. Indeed, the household has functioned as a key site for Jewish practice from its earliest beginnings in Ancient Israel. Archeologists rely almost exclusively upon signs of domestic religiosity—dietary restrictions, concerns for vessel purity, household deities—for evidence of early Israelite presence. Throughout time, and varying from region to region, Jewish households acquired a set of distinctive religious and cultural features that shaped the cycles of work and rest, food preparation and consumption, patterns of assembly and socialization, childrearing, storytelling, song, study, and speech. These practices always displayed regional and temporal variations and were inevitably inflected by specific social, cultural, and linguistic factors. Nevertheless, at the center of Jewish practice lay the household, a key institution of Jewish life from its inception. Indeed, as the present essay will now suggest, not only was the household a central domain for Jewish practice, it functioned as a significant point of origin for customs that were later authorized in rabbinic halakha.

In asserting that the household was a point of origin for customs later formalized in halakha, this essay inverts the more typical depiction of the relationship between household and halakha. For the purposes of discussion, let us consider three typologies in the portrayal of this relationship. The first is perhaps the most traditional: halakha dictates household practice. According to this approach, halakha is a schema of practices systematized by rabbinic figures after the destruction of the Temple, who, through sustained attention to oral traditions, customs, and biblical materials, formulated a way of life that became normative for Jews in late antiquity and beyond. According to this approach, the household was shaped by rabbinic prescription. The second approach considers the household as an alternative domain, a site characterized by folk culture and cross-cultural developments. According to this approach, household folkways developed independently from rabbinic authority, and at times, even at odds with it. A third and final approach identifies the household as a generative domain in the formation of halakha itself. That is, household practices yielded the traditional forms later systematized in rabbinic halakha. The present essay works with this last position, while also blending in elements of the second approach—that is, that the household is a site that operates according to its own vital mode of cultural production. My working theory is that Jewish norms, halakha chief among them, emerge from the dialectical interplay between common Jewish practice and elite, rabbinic formulations. This approach maintains the alterity of the household as a site distinct from rabbinic scholarly circles, but nevertheless, as one that informed rabbinic developments.

A genealogy of halakha that begins in the household corrects for the tendency to narrate the development of Judaism from one set of elite canonical texts to the next. Such accounts are not only too restrictive, leaving out all manner of religious living that did not find its way to the pages of the Bible or the Talmud, but they also tend to be accompanied by a notion that Jewish history is marked by a series of ruptures that are repaired by the ingenuity of elites who formulate new, viable modes of religious practice after older paradigms have worn thin. When one introduces the household into a genealogy of halakha, threads of continuity between a millennium of common Jewish practice and late-antique rabbinic formulations emerge; many of the halakhic practices canonized in rabbinic literature already bore a centuries-long history as common Jewish custom. Indeed, one way to account for the strong reception of rabbinic halakha among late-antique and medieval Jewry was the degree to which a significant portion of its dictates derived from known Jewish practice. Despite the critical-historical assumptions of this essay, therefore, the present emphasis upon the household in the formation of halakha recovers a rather traditional notion of continuity in Jewish practice. It suggests that traditional Jewish practices, while certainly changing and evolving over time, nevertheless have origins as ancient as the people itself.

What evidence can we adduce with regard to the role of the household and its web of social relations in the formation of rabbinic halakha? The integration of household custom into rabbinic prescription was not always a smooth one; we therefore find Talmudic passages that disclose the fraught procedure by which household norms were accommodated and systematized in rabbinic literature. In the pages that follow, we shall trace what Charlotte Fonrobert has called ruptures in the text, instances in which one finds disturbances "in the androcentric fabric" of Talmudic discourse.[3] The assimilation of household custom—often the domain of women's activity and authority—into rabbinic law sometimes proved challenging, and close readings of rabbinic texts reveal a tense interplay between these two realms.

Let us begin with Shabbat. Shabbat provides a fantastic window into the role of the household in shaping halakha, as there is no doubt that Shabbat had a long life in ancient Israel, and in later Jewish society, well before the rabbis systematized its regulations. Let us examine what has become an iconic Shabbat practice: the kindling of lights before the onset of Shabbat. This particular practice was likely to have originated in the necessary household task of ensuring sufficient light for household work and leisure after sunset. The practical measure of lighting lamps produced a custom that, in some ways, became even more significant than the custom of reciting *kiddush* and Torah verses to sanctify the day. The Mishnah assumes the binding nature of this custom, though it would acquire a formal blessing only in the medieval period, perhaps in response to Karaite challenges. The lighting of Shabbat candles, therefore, is an example of household task turned halakhic duty.

Similarly, the two loaves of bread that are a central feature of the Shabbat table are likely to have originated in the household task of preparing double portions on Friday given the prohibitions regarding food prepa-

---

[3] Charlotte Fonrobert, "Yalta's Ruse: Resistance against Rabbinic Menstrual Authority in Talmudic Literature" in Rahel Wasserfall ed., *Women and Water, Menstruation in Jewish Life and Law* (Hanover, NH: Brandeis University Press, 1999), 75.

ration on Shabbat itself. I introduce the household origins of these two important symbolic elements of Shabbat—candle-lighting and the double portion of bread—not to sully sacred Jewish rituals with household origins, but instead to suggest that the very distinction between household operations and sacred tasks may need to be re-examined. I invite the reader to consider any number of household activities that may have followed this same trajectory from household task to religious duty. Food preparation and household work include elements that are constitutive of the religious experience; these household elements sometimes generated what later becomes formal prescription.

Another example of the mutually informing relationship between household and halakha can be found in the instance of the Shabbat *eruv*. The *eruv* is a rabbinic construct that creates a temporary common domain for the purposes of carrying objects from one place to another on Shabbat. In her recent scholarship, Charlotte Fonrobert has identified the way in which the *eruv* is more than just a work-around for the prohibition of carrying objects on Shabbat; the *eruv* presents a rabbinic theory of the neighborhood and of social relations more broadly.[4] Building on Fonrobert's work, I would like add an aspect to our understanding of the *eruv*, namely, that while the *eruv* was a rabbinic invention, the rabbis did not invent the neighborhoods that they authorized. To use a spatial metaphor, here so appropriate, the map of the rabbinic *eruv* corresponded to existing patterns of human circulation and not the reverse.

For example, the courtyard *eruv* involves a collectively designated ritual food item that declares a courtyard and its surrounding households to be a common domain. The *eruv* did not invent the patterns of circulation among these dwellings, but rather reconciles the prohibition of carrying with necessary movement among these households. The courtyard *eruv* gave license to household comings and goings, food sharing, the transportation of objects, and the passage of children. This movement could hardly come to a halt on the Sabbath. It could therefore only come under the canopy of rabbinic governance through the sweeping license of *eruv*.

---

[4] Charlotte Fonrobert, "Gender Politics in the Rabbinic Neighborhood: Tractate Eruvin," in Tal Ilan, Tamara Or, Dorothea M. Salzer, Christiane Steuer and Irina Wandrey, eds., *A Feminist Commentary on the Babylonian Talmud, Introduction and Studies* (Tübingen: Mohr Siebeck, 2007), 44.

To be sure, the Talmud does not admit to the power of household operations in forcing the hand of halakhic reasoning. As Fonrobert notes, "in the entire tractate in the Bavli [Babylonian Talmud], there are only three short Aramaic case-stories…that illustrate what one might need to carry outside of the private domain, and all three involve the scenario of a circumcision coinciding with Shabbat."[5] The Talmud, therefore, presents the *eruv* as an accommodation of the rare instance of the infant whose water has spilt on circumcision day. I would suggest, however, that this unlikely instance stands in for the entire array of activities—unceasing and unnamed—that go on in household life and that required wholesale license of the *eruv* if such functions were to be assimilated into the rabbinic rubric.

The above examples illustrate the process by which a rapprochement was achieved between everyday household operations and halakha. At the same time, other texts indicate even greater strain in the relationship between household operations and rabbinic jurisdiction. The example that I would like to discuss draws from the famous and troubling lines in Mishnah Shabbat:

> For three transgressions women die in childbirth: for neglecting the laws of *niddah* [menstruation], of *hallah* [bread] and of the kindling of [Shabbat and festival] lights. (Shabbat 2:6)

Much can be said about this mishnah and its ominous threat of death in childbirth. It transforms a tragic circumstance into punishment for the neglect of Jewish precepts. Classically, it is read as an indication of the profound patriarchal character of the rabbinic project. I would concur; however, I would also suggest that the uncharacteristic, punitive rhetoric of this mishnah indicates that something more is at play. Rather than a show of rabbinic power over women's ritual practice, the deviant rhetoric of this mishnah in fact indicates weak rabbinic jurisdiction regarding activities over which women served as authorities: menstruation (*niddah*), food preparation (*challah*) and household Shabbat law. As further indication of this, note the uncharacteristic rhetorical frame of the next

---

[5] Fonrobert, "Gender Politics," 46.

mishnah as well:

> Three statements must be made by a person [in or upon
> entering] his home on the eve of Shabbat upon [the fall of]
> darkness: Have you tithed? Have you established an *eruv*;
> **Light the candles!** (Shabbat 2:7)

This is yet another unusual rabbinic exposition: the male head of household enters the domestic setting and delivers a series of declarations in order to enforce *halakhot* related to food and Sabbath preparation. The final command to light the candles is so harsh that the Gemara, as well as later classical medieval commentators, soften the tone of the mishnah by adding: *b'nahat* (gently). I would suggest that this roster of declarations, like the looming threat in the previous mishnah, indicate the *distance* between male, rabbinic authority and these activities. The rhetorical deviance of these two *mishnayot* reveal a disturbance in the rabbinic project in its effort to preside over household functions that operated independently of rabbinic supervision.

Indeed, at the conclusion of this section of the Talmud we encounter a provocative alternative to our mishnah:

> For three sins women die in childbirth… Rav Aha says, for the
> transgression of laundering the filth of their children [diapers]
> on Shabbat. (b. Shabbat, 32a)

What a strange retelling of the more familiar, principal mishnah. This text presents the outrageous pairing of dirty diapers with divine wrath. What is the problem with dirty diapers? How could they provoke such terrible punishment? If the true prompt for the grasping rhetoric of this series of rabbinic statements is the authority of the household and the women who preside there, then this teaching begins to make sense. Dirty diapers present a perfect challenge to the rabbinic claim of total jurisdiction over human life. This basic element of household life—dirty diapers—signals that there are some household tasks that present a major, and perhaps insurmountable, challenge to the halakhic framework. How did one prevent the household from smelling of feces and urine? By washing the diapers, of course. Could such an activity be permitted? Apparently it could not. We have hit the limit of rabbinic license and we are in diaper trouble. The problem of dirty diapers—which may stand in for other household work that cannot be suspended for the 24 hours of Shabbat— undermines the totalizing claim of the rabbinic system.

Why couldn't this element of human activity be redeemed within a schema of rabbinic license? Why couldn't something as basic and necessary as dirty diapers be assimilated into a halakhic framework, much as the *eruv* assimilated pre-existing practice? One might be tempted to attribute this limitation to rabbinic avoidance of human waste, as if feces are too grotesque to be integrated into the laws of Shabbat. Rabbinic law, however, is not squeamish about bodily functions; bodily secretions are treated in great detail throughout the Talmud. I believe that it is the temporal aspect of waste management that poses the greatest challenge to the rabbinic framework. It is not the periodic grotesque that challenges the rabbinic framework, but the constant and necessary work involved in waste management. Consider, by contrast, the ease with which the handling of blood—that is, saving a human life—is addressed in the halakhic system. Perhaps unlike feces, blood represents the loftier element of the human condition; it correlates to the soul and its preservation warrants the suspension of normal Shabbat demands. Such suspension is intermittent, urgent, and transitory. Feces, however, represent the unceasing demands of the human body as well as other household work that does not permit a Sabbath rest. Dirty diapers may stand in for those aspects of being human that resist ritual alteration. To borrow the Talmudic phrase used to describe food preparation that is resistant to alterations on festival days, "it is impossible in any other way."[6] Dirty diapers, it seems, was beyond rabbinic reach.

The tension between household and rabbinic authority becomes even more clear in an addendum to our diaper text. Women die in childbirth because they call the *aron ha-kodesh*, the holy ark, "arna," an Aramaic term for ark (b. Shabbat, 32a). This is yet another mysterious statement unless we consider that a vernacular term for a sacred object poses a simi-

---

[6] Babylonian Talmud, Betsah, 30a. See the rich discussion of these materials in Tamara Or, "'Why Don't we say anything to them?' (b. Bes 30a), Women in Massekhet Betsah," in Tal Ilan, et al., *A Feminist Commentary*, 183-196.

lar threat to the totality of the rabbinic claim. The power to name sacred objects, or, as Bourdieu would tell us, the power to produce language of sacred register, is the purview of the religious establishment and not the populace. The existence of a religious vernacular realm in which items in the synagogue may go by any other name, undermines the total rabbinic claim over Jewish life. Indeed, just after this statement, another teaching appears in which the competition between household vernacular and rabbinic issue is made explicit. In this next statement, the transgression of using a vernacular term is attributed to commoners/ignoramuses (*amei ha'aratzot*). They too have coined a Jewish term, and that is their fatal sin: they are struck down by God for the sin of calling the *beit knesset* (house of assembly), a *beit am* (house of the people). These texts, and perhaps this entire set of troubled texts in Tractate Shabbat, reveal a tension between vernacular renderings and rabbinic articulations. These fissures in the text, however, do not reveal the unassimilable relationship between household and halakha, but quite the reverse. They reveal the potent and living interplay between common custom and rabbinic conversation.

The present analysis of the household origins of halakha draws its theoretical underpinnings from the highly influential paper by Haym Soloveitchik, "Rupture and Reconstruction, the Transformation of Contemporary Orthodoxy," a paper that forever changed how traditional Jewish life would be understood.[7] In this paper, Soloveitchik argued that the mimetic process by which halakha was formed and transmitted in previous eras—a blend of rabbinic precedent and common Jewish practice—has been replaced by a text-based procedure that grants little if any religious authority to communal habits and practice. Halakha is now arbitrated through consultation with rabbinic texts alone and traditional behaviors, "once governed by habit," are now "governed by rule."[8] Soloveitchik's article reached a wide audience, from popular readers who were curious about the developments they were experiencing firsthand, to historians who began to use his analytical categories to examine previous phases of Jewish cultural production. Soloveitchik's observations became so commonplace that his categories of mimetic vs. text-based processes began to appear

---

[7] Haym Soloveitchik, "Rupture and Reconstruction, the Transformation of Contemporary Orthodoxy," in Tradition, a Journal of Orthodox Jewish Thought (1994; 28:4): 64-130

[8] Soloveitchik, 71.

without any reference to the article itself. This I take as the best evidence of the immediate resonance that his analysis has adduced.

Throughout his essay, Soloveitchik uses the term "kitchen apprentice-ship" to capture the broader process of mimetic transmission and its various domains: the kitchen, yes, but also the household, the street, the storefront, the *shul*. The kitchen is shorthand for all of these informal, non-text-based environments that played a formative role in the halakhic formations of previous eras. Modernity has weakened these many sites of Jewish cultural production, but it has not destroyed them.

We now find ourselves in a time of pandemic and all that remains is the kitchen. Despite its weakened authority in the modern age, the kitchen has retained its extraordinary importance in Jewish practice, and this im-portance is now intensified in the pandemic. Traditional Jewish practices can unfold in even the most isolated of households. The smallest ritual gesture can introduce a reflective and even beautiful quality to our lives. The utterance of a short blessing, the preparation of a family recipe, the lighting of a candle, the sweeping out of one's pantry—any one of these actions can introduce a meditative reckoning with the fragility, beauty and inter-dependence of our human lives. Throughout Jewish history, domestic activity formed a context within which one could continue the habits of Jewish life, even in the most trying of circumstances. These hab-its include with whom one associated, how one prepared foods, and the style in which one fed and soothed one's children. The household was the principal matrix for the development of Jewish practice over time. Our current crisis, therefore, does not take us beyond the terms of halakhic development itself. Something new will emerge in the circumstances of this pandemic, but the household as the defining site of Jewish living has a long history, to which we are now adding a chapter.

Community, Solidarity, and Love
in the Time of Covid-19

Ariel Evan Mayse

Rabbinic Judaism was born of a crucible, emerging in the aftermath of the Temple's destruction. The pages of the Talmud and the classical *midrashim* are filled with haunting descriptions of communal devastation and personal tragedy, and rabbinic sages and later commentators grappled with explaining how, and why, God might allow such suffering to transpire.[1] Many of these hardships, though perceived to be divine in origin, emerge from physical phenomena rooted in the natural world. The teachings included in b. Ta'anit—a tractate exploring the contours of fast days decreed in response to drought, famine, and plague—offer a particularly vivid vocabulary for considering the earthshattering impact of Covid-19 and the social, economic, and theological crises born in its wake.[2] Its teachings raise enduring questions regarding human agency and empowerment engendered by these tragedies. And they present both a ritualized fabric and an ethos of communal solidarity as central to the response to communal or global suffering

Noting a number of tentative reasons why rain might be withheld,[3] the tractate opens with a vigorous reminder that human power is indeed limited: "Three keys are held by the blessed Holy One that have not been delivered to a messenger, and these are they: the keys of rain, of the childbearing woman, and of resurrection."[4] When rain does come, either simply by heavenly fiat or in response to human prayer and fasting, the day is recalled as a momentous occasion akin to the world's creation or the

---

[1] See b. Berakhot 5a-b; b. Hagigah 5a-b; b. Gittin 55b-57a; and the stories recounted in Eikhah Rabbah.

[2] I wish to express gratitude Dr. Deena Aranoff, Dr. Melila Hellner-Eshed and Professor Menachem Lorberbaum, teachers with whom I have had the privilege of studying b. Ta'anit for many years.

[3] b. Ta'anit 7a-8a.

[4] b. Ta'anit 2a.

giving of the Torah.[5] An acute sense of collective destiny thus undergirds this vision of the life-giving power of rain. Rabbi Eliezer says, "The entire world is sustained by the waters of the ocean," and Rabbi Yehoshua says, "It is sustained by the supernal waters," a disagreement that nonetheless reveals a shared belief that all human beings depend on common (or shared) resources to which access is not entirely in our control.[6] These rabbinic discussions reflect an awareness that such phenomena, like weather patterns, are not simply a local matter. Plagues can easily extend beyond their initial ground zero, and the debilitating ripple effects of drought stop at neither individual nor communal borders. The proper response to the impact of these tragedies, suggest the rabbis in Ta'anit, demands both social solidarity as well as individual action.

The series of fasts decreed when rains are dangerously delayed begins with certain elect persons (called *yehidim*) refraining from food and drink.[7] They represent, in a sense, the spiritual vanguard who take the suffering of the many upon themselves when tragedy appears upon the horizon. Although the majority of the tractate is concerned with public fasts, many teachings in Ta'anit highlight each and every individual's responsibility to contribute toward communal solidarity. One who travels from a non-fasting community to a location in which people are fasting must fast with his new neighbors.[8] An individual who has forgotten that he should be fasting together with his community and mistakenly eats or drinks should not, claims the Talmud, eat in front of others, nor can he comport himself by enjoying delightful foods.[9] In Rashi's felicitous rendering, by doing so one "appears as a bridegroom among mourners." Later scholars understand this prohibition against special foods as applying even if one is alone—the individual's indulgence is utterly problematic even if it is hidden away within the private domain. This suggests that the moral concern here is not only for the appearance of non-compliance, but with the ethical flaccidity and lack of solidarity of one who revels in merriment while those immediately around him are suffering.

The active response is solidarity, of holding together in the face of crisis.

---

[5] b. Ta'anit 7a-b.
[6] b. Ta'anit 9b.
[7] m. Ta'anit 1:4.
[8] b. Ta'anit 10b.
[9] Ibid.

This posture is summed up nicely in a series of teachings that function as a kind of ethical scaffolding for much of the tractate:

> Rabbi Yehudah said in the name of Rav: One who starves himself during years of famine is saved from a strange death, as it says, "He will redeem you from death with famine." (Job 5:20)

By reading be-ra'av as "with" or "by means of famine" rather than "from famine," Rabbi Yehudah suggests that voluntary acts of supererogatory piety prevent famine from reaching one's own doorstep. There appears to be more than a vestige of self-interest in this practice, since one's purpose in giving up food is self-preservation. But the next statement is even bolder.

> Resh Lakish said: It is forbidden for one to engage in sexual relations during a time of famine, as it says, "And two sons were born to Joseph before the year of famine came." (Gen. 41:50)

Perhaps this expression of volitional suffering (abstaining from sexual relations) is construed as having some penitential impact on God. Perhaps, however, the essential point is that the suffering must be willingly undertaken in order to express solidarity with a weakened community, to cultivate compassion and to performatively embody empathy. Conjugal relations are forbidden during times of acute suffering, according to one reading of Resh Lakish's statement, because focusing on such personal, intimate delight diminishes one's attunement to the suffering of others. Conscious engagement with the other people's pain is necessary even if one can, in theory, remain untouched by the drought or the plague.

Such is the implication of the next series of statements, which moves the threshold of suffering to one's immediate spiritual (and perhaps also geographic) community:

> When the Jewish people are in distress and one separates from them, the two ministering angels that accompany a person come and put their hands on his head and say, "This person who has withdrawn from the community will not see it be comforted."...

When the community is immersed in pain, a person may not say: "I will go to my home and I will eat and drink, and peace be upon you, my soul." ... one must suffer along with the community... and one who suffers with the community will merit seeing the consolation of the community.[10]

This is a searing indictment of self-interest in the face of the suffering of other people. Only studied, conscious solidarity—not simply shared commiseration—provides a society with the power to confront human suffering. An individual who does take part in the travails of his or her world cannot enjoy the future consolation; one cannot really be a part of the redemption if one has not been party to the sufferings of exile. And perhaps the Talmud means to suggest something more: solidarity and unity lead to the community's redemption.

Similar reflections on the power of spiritual solidarity appear as central concerns in the literature of Hasidism, an essentially social form of mystical devotion anchored in charismatic leadership and lived out in intense communal life. Hasidic texts maintain that personal religious journeys are fundamentally intertwined with the lives of others, and its teachings have much to offer our world in which societal fabrics are being brutally torn apart and endemic racism exposed.

Rabbi Yisra'el of Kozhentis (1737-1814), for example, sermonically deploying the *Shulchan Arukh's* rule that the quorum (*minyan*) must be in a single place, notes that "All ten [individuals of the quorum] must be 'in one place'—directing themselves toward the Cosmic One, praying that He and His name will be one, that God's kingdom will soon be revealed to us."[11] Jewish sources, including those of b. Ta'anit, have long emphasized the efficacy of communal prayer and shared religious gestures. Hasidism takes this a step further, arguing that the participants must comprise a group unified toward a spiritual goal rather than a diffuse assembly of individuals.

Some Hasidic sources emphasize that, in times of duress, we are to connect ourselves to spiritual teachers or leaders. The *rebbe* or *tsaddik*, a combination of rabbi, shaman, prophet, king, and priest,[12] is said to serve

---

[10] b. Ta'anit 11a.

[11] Ariel Evan Mayse and Sam Berrin Shonkoff, eds., *Hasidism: Writings on Devotion, Community and Life in the Modern World* (Waltham: Brandeis University Press, 2020), 94–95.

[12] Arthur Green, "Typologies of Leadership and the Hasidic Zaddiq," *Jewish Spirituality II: From the Sixteenth-Century Revival to the Present*, ed. A. Green (New York: Crossroad, 1987), 127-156; idem, "The Zaddiq as Axis Mundi," 327-347.

as a conduit for divine compassion and blessing who cannot abide the suffering of others:

> They are connected to the Creator's attributes, including abundant compassion, and they cannot bear to see any Jew in any sort of suffering, God forbid! They seek compassion upon all [and for each] individual, which is God's will… People who conduct themselves in this manner may interrupt the study of Torah, or other kinds of communion with God or the healing of their [own] souls. There are others, however, who are interested only in preparing their own souls.[13]

Some accomplished talents seek only to perfect their own spiritual progress, but true spiritual guides and teachers must display deep pathos, compassion, and concern for their followers. The ideal of Hasidic leadership is defined not by isolated intellectual or spiritual achievement, but by empowering and ennobling all those to whom the teacher is connected. Such leaders become fulcra of solidarity, a courageous source of support to the devotional community that crystallizes around them.

Hasidism puts great stock in horizontal relationships between fellow travelers, especially in times of duress. This quality of *dibbuk chaverim*, or connection among spiritual friends, was upheld as a cardinal value. "Each person should see to it that he has a regular practice of spiritual friendship with those he knows well, who are trusted and committed to the truth alone," writes Rabbi Menachem Mendel of Vitsebsk (1730-1788). "These companions should share in your yearning to loosen the fetters of evil— that is, the desires of hypocrisy and falsehood."[14] This powerful emphasis on mutuality, solidarity, love, and friendship as the ground of all spiritual growth has much to teach us in a world that is fractious, balkanized, and torn.[15] This call to assemble and connect—as Jewish communities often beset with infighting, but also as civically-engaged members of a polarized American people—invites us toward healing even across difference.

But what happens when things fall apart? Here we turn to the writings

---

[13] From Zot Zikaron, translated in Mayse and Shonkoff, *Hasidism*, 97.

[14] Mayse and Shonkoff, *Hasidism*, 62.

[15] On neo-Hasidic visions of such intentional communities, see Arthur Green and Ariel Evan Mayse, eds., *A New Hasidism: Roots* (Philadelphia: Jewish Publication Society, 2019), esp. 1-50, and Ebn Leader's essay "Does a New Hasidism Need Rebbes?" in idem, *A New Hasidism: Branches*, 317-338.

of Rabbi Kalonymous Kalman Shapira (1889 -1943), better known as the *Esh Kodesh* or the Rebbe of the Warsaw Ghetto. The idea of community is a major theme in his early writings, and in the 1920s Shapira wrote a short pamphlet entitled *Beney Mahashavah Tovah*, best translated as "children of a heightened (or intensified) consciousness," to outline the basic principles and structures of a close-knit mystical fellowship. Shapira's wartime sermons are also filled with stirring reflections on spiritual community forged in mutuality and reciprocity:

> [The angels are described] as "receiving one from the other" (*mekablin dein min dein*).[16] We receive from one another not only when we give *tsedakah* or other kinds of love to each other, but also when one listens to the suffering of another Jew and does all that can be done to help, if his heart is shattered within and the blood freezes up in his veins, and if from this broken heart he returns to God and prays to the blessed One on behalf of Israel. This, too, is a kind of receiving "one from the other"— he receives brokenheartedness and repentance, and they, from him, [receive] compassion, good deeds and prayer performed on their behalf. This causes [the angels] on high to receive from one another.[17]

In this beautiful description of theurgic empathy, the angelic chorus is said to mirror acts of human compassion down below. This includes generosity manifest in concrete deeds, but Shapira is highlighting the binding power of dialogue and the present, engaged solidarity expressed through the art of listening to and participating in the suffering of the other. The listener receives a measure of transformative brokenheartedness, and the speaker receives acts of love in addition to a listening ear. Thus do the angelic wings begin to flutter and erupt in liturgical song, filling the cosmos with yet another measure of mercy and illumination. To borrow from Portia, the quality of mercy, it seems, is quite literally twice blessed.

The noted theologian and scholar Howard Thurman once argued that the truest form of love for the other, a posture and disposition cultivated through a rich mystical life of interiority, is "intrinsic interest in another

---

[16] Recited as part of the morning liturgy.

[17] Kalonymous Kalman Shapira, *Derashot mi-Shenot ha-Za'am*, ed. Daniel Reiser, 2 vols. (Jerusalem: Herzog Academic College, 2017), vol. 1, 112.

person for his own sake."[18] "Men do not love in general," wrote Thurman, "but they do love in particular. To love means dealing with persons in the concrete rather than in the abstract."[19] The expressions of love and solidarity that we must cultivate toward those around us will remain weak and impoverished as long as it is abstract and intransitive. We must, demands Thurman, come to appreciate both the inner beauty and the multifaceted complexity and specificity of each and every person in our world. Only thus can we appreciate the fullness of who they are and, when times require it, link arms and stand in solidarity for a common goal.

Covid-19 will not be stopped just by openheartedness or recognizing the inner beauty in others, but its impact and aftermath can be shaped through shared intention and commitment to shared communal destiny. The pandemic has highlighted the systemic racism of our country and its staggeringly disproportionate impact upon communities of color and individuals of fragile or less privileged socioeconomic status. The Kotsker Rebbe (1787-1859) is said to have quipped, "I am not afraid of war, but I am terrified of how people behave in its wake." This truism might just as well apply to the current pandemic. The devastating mortality of the disease is tragedy enough, but its imbalanced impact is all the more cruel. The pandemic has revealed the tremendous iniquities and inequalities of American society, and, rather than returning to "normalcy," we must seize this opportunity to dramatically rethink our economic and social structures.

A response to this crisis founded in communal solidarity requires that we, as Jews, reappraise who we do--and do not—include within our circles of solidarity. It has become de rigueur to quote Abraham Joshua Heschel's biting and beloved aphorism "In a free society, some are guilty. All are responsible." As American citizens, we are indeed responsible parties in racial and economic injustice that have been further exacerbated by Covid-19, and that may be putting it too lightly. Indifference, argued both Heschel and Elie Wiesel, is the true inverse of the good. The antidote to xenophobia, rhetoric of division, and demonization is found in a call for nuance, patient presence, empathy, truly seeing the position of others, and recognizing that we have been, thus far, complicit and even guilty. This point has been driven home by educator and entrepreneur Yavilah McCoy, who writes:

---

[18] Howard Thurman, *Mysticism and the Experience of Love* (Wallingford, PA: Pendle Hill, 1961), 12.

[19] Ibid, 13.

During Covid-19, a veil was lifted for my staff and the POC/JOC [People of Color/Jews of Color] community we serve that revealed just how commoditized and expendable women of colors' bodies are in a racialized system that consistently devalues our worth and teaches us to only value ourselves in the context of services we can provide for a White majority...

In our work, we are encountering smart, brilliant, high performing Jewish people of color who are describing being exhausted at the prospect of continuing to deliver their labor within systems that erase us.[20]

Solidarity is meaningful to the extent that it includes *all* of the people in our community, acknowledging that diversity and intersectional identities need not undermine such efforts. McCoy has laid forth a challenge, seeking "partners in Jewish spaces who see our liberation as their liberation and who will work with us to deepen opportunities for wellness and greater equity for all of us." This is an important call to which we must rise, realizing that the freedom of the collective depends upon the freedom of each and every member.

A Hasidic teaching from Rabbi Zeev Wolf of Zhitomir (d. 1800), who notes that Egypt was struck by a plague of shadow so thick that "people did not see their companions and no person could rise from where he was seated" (Ex. 10: 23), speaks to this point:

"See" means that they didn't consider them ... they didn't take to heart how much they could learn from the goodness of the people around them. On the contrary, they kept finding fault and lack in others, glorifying their own deeds. This led them to walk about in darkness and to see no light. People like that cannot progress from one rung to the next; "no person could rise from where he was seated." They stood about rather than walking forward, as a Jew is always supposed to do.[21]

[20] Yavilah McCoy, "Dancing between Light and Shadow—Increasing Awareness of the Impact of Covid-19 Disparities on Jews of Color," eJewish Philanthropy (May 21, 2020), accessible at: https://ejewishphilanthropy.com/dancing-between-light-and-shadow-increasing-awareness-of-the-impact-of-covid-19-disparities-on-jews-of-color/, accessed July 12, 2020.

[21] Or ha-Me'ir, translated in Arthur Green, *Speaking Torah: Spiritual Teachings from Around the Maggid's Table*, with Ebn Leader, Ariel Evan Mayse and Or N. Rose (Woodstock, VT:

Our own spiritual development is stalled when we deny the necessity of learning from everyone in our community. To be sure, turning to witness the pain and suffering around us will be discomforting. We must, however, come to see the people whose voices are suppressed, who are hidden and ignored, whose humanity is denied and denigrated at every turn. One must engage in such struggles for liberation with the understanding that this is not *their* problem, but *our* problem as well.

This important point returns us to another dimension of b. Ta'anit, one that is particularly visible in the tales of mysterious wonder-workers, pious individuals and sages who populate the third chapter of the tractate. Many of the characters and personalities who appear in this chapter, and are really its heart, are manifestations of tensions and problems which emerge from key themes in the entire tractate. It is surely no accident that this chapter has so many strange characters within a tractate that is otherwise focused on creating norms and order. Perhaps nowhere is this driven home with more power than in the story of Rabbi Eliezer whose "head was swollen with pride because he had studied much Torah." This hubris leads him to callously insult another person,[22] and although he is shielded somewhat because of his erudition, Rabbi Eliezer's haughtiness—that of untrammeled elitist pride—is condemned. "One must always be as soft as a reed," he pronounces, "and not stiff like a cedar." Supple humility rather than rigid hubris allows one to see that Torah comes from everywhere in the world, even or especially from those places most on the margins.

Covid-19 has shown us that our world, globalized and local, is fractured with inequality. Solidarity in the face of the pandemic demands that we confront uncomfortable truths about our complicity and guilt in economic and racial oppression. This experience has also shown us that our worlds must grow to include the critical teachings of those who have been largely ignored. The power of Torah is expanded and enriched by new teachings of liberation, emancipation, and empowerment—as well as hermeneutical and theological legacies forged in suffering, pain, and reclamation. "One who suffers with the community," asserts the Talmud, "will merit witnessing its consolation."[23] By standing together to face the consequences of Covid-19, we begin the healing work of expanding our Torah and walking the path of compassion.

Jewish Lights Publications, 2013), vol. 1, 184.
   [22] b. Ta'anit 20a–b
   [23] b. Ta'anit 11a.

Building an Ark in the Midst of a Flood:
Mindfulness Practices for Staying Afloat

James Jacobson-Maisels

We are living in an overwhelming time brought on by both a plague and a host of social and political upheavals which have disrupted our daily lives, upended our institutions, crashed our economies, and caused devastating losses of lives. In the face of these unfolding crises, many of us feel overwhelmed, like it's all just too much. Too much uncertainty, too much to handle, too many demands, too many emotions, too much pressure, too many thoughts, too many decisions, too many people in one small house, too much isolation, and too much fear.

This "too much" feeling is familiar to many of us. Yet at a moment when this feeling is so intense, how do we stay clear and connected to ourselves, one another, and the Divine? How do we not give in to fear? How do we act responsibly to protect ourselves and others and bring transformation and change without getting lost in despair or desperation or falling into complacency?

While the Covid-19 pandemic may feel unprecedented to us, this degree of uncertainty and vulnerability, the sense of overwhelm, was not foreign to our ancestors. Indeed, it was once an assumed part of human life. Our ancestors faced plagues, expulsions, wars, and upheavals, and used the wisdom of their Judaism to meet those daunting challenges. In that tradition, I want to present here some of the ways the Jewish tradition has given us to cope with the overwhelm that we can feel in such moments.

Mayim Rabim—The Flood

One of the most powerful images of overwhelm in our texts can be found in Psalm 32: "Therefore let every pious one pray to You, when he is found, that the rushing mighty waters (*mayim rabim*) not overtake him" (Ps. 32:6). This image of rushing mighty waters, *mayim rabim*, is later taken up in the Hasidic tradition as a way to describe that moment when unwanted and unhelpful thoughts, emotions, and sensations threaten to swamp us, an experience the Hasidic tradition calls *mahshavot zarot* (alien states of consciousness). This image of flooding conveys our internal sense of being lost in a wave of thought or emotion. It recalls that primal biblical image of the flood which threatens "to destroy all flesh which has the breath of life within it" (Gen. 6:17). Indeed, it can feel like "the wellsprings of the vast deep have broken forth and the floodgates of the sky have broken open" (Gen. 2:11). We can be engulfed by a range of emotions (anger, desire, confusion, hurt, anxiety), by the recognition of the basic and profound uncertainty and instability of our world, or by excessive and obsessive thought (rehearsing, fantasy, planning, worrying, fixing). Someone says something that feels hurtful, critical, or threatening, and we are filled with anger, self-blame, or shame. Your boss mentions that the company is in trouble, for example, and the mind starts spinning out of control wondering if you are going to be laid off, what you will do, how you and your family will cope; the chest tightens, the heart speeds up, and there is a sick feeling in the pit of your stomach.

R. Kalonymus Kalmish Shapira, the Piaseczner Rebbe (1889-1943), provides us with three metaphors to describe how we might experience this flood of thought and emotion. Sometimes, he tells us, we feel as if we are caught in a slingshot, flung in all directions, unable to orient ourselves. At other times, we might feel like we're drowning, sinking to the bottom of a swamp. Or we may simply feel so overwhelmed that we shut down. It is as if, he says, piles of garbage have been dumped on top of our soul and heart, smothering our emotions—both joyful feelings and painful ones— or blanketing us in a dulling anxiety.[1] These are all versions of the *mayim rabim*, the great waters, that threaten to overwhelm us, leaving us feeling lost and destabilized.

When we are caught in one of these states, we often have one of three responses: Lashing, Thrashing, or Shutting Down.

When we lash out, we yell, criticize, and blame (ourselves or others), become defensive or spiteful. Our body may become tight, our muscles tense. Our reserves of patience are low. So when our partner does that thing we find annoying, or our child refuses to listen, or our colleague drops the ball on the project due tomorrow, we react, lashing out at them, or fuming and ruminating internally.

At other times we start to thrash, desperately trying to regain control and balance. The Baal Shem Tov (known as the Besht, 1700-1760, the founder of Hasidism) describes an image of a person lost in *mahshavot zarot* (foreign

---

[1] Kalonymus Kalmish Shapira, *Hakhsharat HaAvrekhim, Mevo HaShearim (L'Hovat HaAvrekhim), Tzav VeZeruz.* (Jerusalem: Va'ad Haside Piaseczno (Committee of Piasczno Hasidim), 5761 (2001)), §1, 4-5.

mind states) as one drowning in a river, flailing and thrashing their arms to keep from sinking.[2] We anxiously scroll through news updates on our phones, as if that will somehow make us feel safer and more empowered. Or we become increasingly controlling—with ourselves and everyone around us—desperately trying to make sure everything is taken care of, everything is in order, and everything will be all right. Of course that thrashing, as with the drowning person, is not an effective means of keeping us afloat. But at the moment we don't know what else to do.

Or we shut down. It's all just too much, too overwhelming, so we just stop feeling anything at all. We burrow into that pile of garbage the Piaseczner described. We may feel numb, anxious, depressed, or like we're in a fog or a daze.

So what do we do when we are flooded? The Torah already tells us: We build an ark. We create something that can keep us afloat so we can ride out the waves of the flood. The word for ark in Hebrew, *teivah*, can also mean "word," and the Hasidic masters understood the words of our prayers as the ark which allows us to stay afloat in the midst of the flood.[3]

What spiritual tools and practices might serve as our ark in these challenging times? When we can't find shelter from the storm, how might we attain buoyancy and clarity that allow us to ride out the flood without getting swamped? In the following, I want to introduce four concrete practices from the Jewish tradition and contemporary meditative traditions that can help us build an ark in times of challenge.

Awareness

The first practice is simply that of awareness. The Piaseczner Rebbe teaches that when we bring a powerful embodied awareness to our experience, what he calls *mahshava hazaka*, then we are able to be present, open, and loving with our emotions without getting overwhelmed by them or shutting down.[4] For instance, we have an important project due tomorrow that we don't feel we've done well enough. Anxiety starts to arise in us and feels like it might soon get out of control. One hand moves toward chocolate and the other reaches to turn on some show or see what someone has

---

[2] Israel Baal Shem Tov, ed. J. Immanuel Schochet, *Keter Shem Tov HaShalem* (Brooklyn: Kehot, 2004), 122-123.

[3] R. Ephraim of Sudylkow, *Degel Mahaneh Efrayim*, Noah, d.h. U-Petah. Sefaria: https://www.sefaria.org.il/Degel_Machaneh_Ephraim%2C_Noach?lang=he

[4] Shapira, *Hakhsharat HaAvrekhim*, 31.

posted to dull and distract us from this unpleasant emotion. Yet instead of drowning in the anxiety, we can bring a grounded awareness to the anxiety itself—noticing the racing thoughts, the fluttering in the tummy, the tightness of the chest—and compassionately holding all of that experience in a loving presence as if it were a crying child. Rather than undoing you, this mode of relating stirs compassion and care and grounds you in your own strength and clarity, your ability to be with whatever arises. Rather than turning toward some unhelpful habit to avoid the emotions, you can make clear, non-panicked choices about what, if anything, you should be doing now to make the project better, or whether you have done enough and it is time to let it go until tomorrow.

Standing outside of our experience, we can extend a stick to the part of ourselves that is drowning in the swamp, still the frenetic motion of the slingshot, or gently clear away the garbage pile to allow the tender voice of the soul to come forth. Rather than letting our rising emotions spiral out of control, we can intervene before they overwhelm us—not to shut the emotions down, but rather to open to them with some buoyancy and clarity. This way, what might have become a flood of incapacitating emotions instead becomes a cleansing river, as the Piaseczner describes it,[5] that allows our feelings to simply move through us in a way that is enlivening and liberating.

It is in this sense that the Torah tells us that the ark must have an "opening for the light" (Gen. 6:16). This is precisely what mindfulness does. It lets in some light and air so we can choose other ways of reacting and see something bigger than the flood—the majestic and wide open sky that lets our hearts touch something more expansive. This expansiveness can be a way of connecting with the Divine. For, as the Midrash teaches, "there is no empty space without the presence of the *Shekhinah* (divine presence)" (Exodus Rabba 2:5). When we are able to find our spaciousness again, to rescue ourselves from whatever narrow place is trapping us, even if only for a moment, the Divine is there.

Cultivating Love

A second way to build the ark we need to cope with a flood of overwhelm is to cultivate love. As the Song of Songs teaches us, "Vast floods *(mayim*

---

[5] Shapira, B*nei Mahshavah Tovah* (Jerusalem: Va'ad Haside Piaseczno (Committee of Piaszno Hasidim), 5749 (1989)), 27.

rabim) cannot quench love, nor rivers drown it" (8:7). The idea of using love to anchor ourselves in times of crisis may sound Pollyanna-ish. But think back to a moment when you felt deep love for another person, or felt deeply loved by someone. In that moment, chances are that you felt less overwhelmed by whatever challenges you were facing. Perhaps this is because when we are in touch with love, we feel less isolated and more supported. Or perhaps it is because love is fundamentally grounding, for as the Zohar teaches, "the whole world exists because of love... and all exists through love" (III:267b). When we open to love we are opening to the very nature of reality, the life-force and sap of the universe. Love is the fiber from which the fabric of creation is woven. Held in it we are at home: clear, stable, open, and safe.

We can employ a number of practices to cultivate feelings of love and belovedness. We can repeat certain phrases as part of a meditation such as "may I know that I am loved," or "may you be held in love," as the Piaseczner Rebbe teaches.[6] We can also set aside some time to call to mind each person in our life who has ever shown us love, from the time we were born to the present moment. And not just our closest friends and family members, but our teachers, coaches, neighbors, school bus drivers, colleagues, parents of childhood friends, a random clerk who smiled at us one day, and any others who have shown us care and concern. We can go year by year through our lives, picturing each of these people and remembering how they made us feel, recognizing that we could not have survived our childhood without the care of others. Touching our belovedness not only frees us from the narrow mind and heart but enables us to emerge as our best selves.[7] Or we can, as the blessing before the Shema reminds us, remember that we are held in the "great" and "eternal" Divine love.

The Beauty of the Flood

A third approach to coping with the flood of overwhelm is to recognize the beauty and power of the flood itself, discovering within the waters a precious resource. Indeed, in other places in the Bible the term *mayim rabim* conveys life, power, and beauty, such as when it describes the life-giving water Moses brings forth from the rock (Num. 20:11), or depicts

---

[6] Shapira, *Derekh HaMelekh, Inyan HaShkeitah*, (Jerusalem: Va'ad Haside Piaseczno (Committee of Piasczno Hasidim), 5755 (1995)), 450-451.

[7] Shapira, *Derekh HaMelekh*, Rosh HaShanah 2nd Night 5691, 227-231.

God's voice and angels' wings as sounding like "mighty waters" (Ez. 1:24). Moreover, one of the classic rabbinic images for Torah is water. So while water can take the form of a flood, it can also be the spring, well, or fountain that sustains life itself. The difference is in how we relate to it.

The Piaseczner Rebbe, for instance, explains that our feeling of being overwhelmed often results from how we react to an external circumstance. Instead of viewing whatever is stirring us as a resource, we view it as a threat and immediately resist it:

> Know dear one it is not that we err but rather that the people of the world err in thinking that this world which God created is a kind of storehouse of evil desires, thoughts and inclinations, and that one who wants to serve God must leave and distance himself from the world entirely. Due to this they spend all their days far from spiritual practice and holiness and sunk in the foolishness of the world. They are like one who sees someone drowning himself in a river and declares that water is an evil thing in the world which was created only to kill. How foolish this person is! Can one live without water? Just because this mentally disturbed person did not utilize water properly and instead of using it to give life to vegetation, animals and people killed himself with it, is it evil?![8]

As R. Shapira notes, while the river is a danger to one who cannot swim, water is also necessary for that person's survival, so rejecting water entirely is not a wise response. But many of us do some version of this in our own lives. For instance, hurt by a relationship, we may pull away from intimacy and trust altogether, robbing ourselves of core human contact, support, and interaction crucial to our flourishing. Instead, we can see the beauty and power of intimacy and our deep yearning for connection, while lovingly embracing the loss and sadness that such connection can bring, and use that to open, heal, and reconnect the heart.

How do we do this? By opening to our fullness. When we enter the ark, we bring everything inside. The Torah tells us that Noah is told to bring "two of every living thing" into the ark (Gen. 6:19), on which Rashi comments, "Every living thing—This means even demons." We can welcome

---

[8] Shapira, *Hovat HaTalmidim* (Tel Aviv: Va'ad Haside Piaseczno (Committee of Piasczno Hasidim), undated), 136.

in the fear, anger, hurt, critique, threat, defensiveness, and whatever else may be arising and have them become an opportunity for healing. The ark is not an escape from grief and pain, but rather a way to hold them in the vastness of both the ocean and the sky. We are saved from the flood, or the wild animals of our emotions, not by shutting the doors on them but by welcoming them in with love. When they are welcomed, we are transformed. The waters are no longer a flood but rather a resource, a vital force that helps make up the wholeness of life.

Exploring Safety, Fear, and Support

A fourth practice for dealing with overwhelm is to explore our experience and understanding of safety so we might find support in difficult times. Safety is a fundamental human need. And we all experience being unsafe in different ways and to different extents, informed by our particular circumstances or identities.

When we or others are unsafe, we should of course do what we can—personally, communally, and politically—to make our and others' lives as safe as possible. Yet whether external change is possible or not in any particular moment, certain forms of practice and ways of thinking that I will describe below may be able to make us feel more supported.

It is perhaps obvious why the question of safety would be especially important to explore in a time of plague and profound instability. In particular, the sense of overwhelm we have been describing often results from a feeling of being unsafe. During this challenging time, we may sit in our house uncertain whether we and our loved ones will be safe from the plague and uncertain whether we will keep our jobs and be able to support ourselves and our families. Or we may be out in the streets protesting, fearful of being met with violence and uncertain of our physical safety. Or we may be experiencing whatever our normal challenges are and the sense of instability they bring up. In addition, all of these various challenges are in dialogue with our own history, constitution, experiences, and habits of response. This means that our perception of threat or lack of safety may not be accurate, whether over- or under- estimating the danger.

Our response to this sense of threat is often to desperately try to find safety. At times, this can be the logical and reasonable thing to do, such as when we are under physical attack. At other times, this sense of desperation does not serve us and we can respond more wisely and effectively if we can create some space around the fear. Perhaps, for instance, worries about your job and financial security have arisen; surely a reasonable concern at this moment. But you may also notice that the anxiety it produces does not actually serve you in getting as clear as you can about the potential threat to your livelihood. Perhaps there are other ways of responding that could serve you better in the face of this and other challenges? All of the practices we have already mentioned can help support us in finding some stability in the midst of such a storm, but I want to suggest some other approaches to the issues of safety in particular that can be helpful.

The first approach is to try to find whatever safety we can in this moment—to build for ourselves an ark. One way to do that is somatically or sensorially. Much of the time, most of our emotions are felt between our waist and head and are wrapped up in cycles of thought. When we are fearful or anxious, the somatic experience of that may be a tightness in the chest, a queasiness in the stomach, or a tension in the face—and it may be accompanied by racing thoughts or disturbing images. When we shift our attention from these experiences to the elbow, the inside of the knee, the feet on the floor or to our bottom on the chair—places in our body which generally feel either neutral or actually rooted and grounded and therefore more supportive—we can start to feel a sense of stability. Similarly, we might bring our attention to a pleasant or supportive sensation, whether in the body, in our external sensory experience, or in our imagination or memory. In all of these cases, focusing on these parts of our experience allows us to resist the pull of the fear vortex that may be arising elsewhere in our body and mind. It can give us some sense of relief, some separation from the fear cycle in our system, so that we might productively find our grounding.

Another way to do this is cognitively. We might ask ourselves questions like: Right now, do I have shelter? Do I have food and water? Do I have clothing? Am I physically safe right now? Asking these questions in situations where the answer is *yes*, or *yes for right now*, or *as far as I know, yes*, can help us recognize that we are safe in a basic existential sense *at this moment*, even when parts of ourselves feel unsafe and/or are unsafe. This realization can start to calm us down and help us feel less panicked and more able to respond wisely.

Doing this can help us touch a broader sense of safety or support that is not as dependent on external circumstances. This, I think, is the meaning of "Israel trusts in God who is their Help and Defender" (Ps. 115:19), or what it might mean to have faith. I don't mean that we trust that God will make everything turn out okay, as that is clearly not true. Anyone who has lived a human life knows that not everything turns out okay. Rather, this trust or faith might be an experience of grounding myself in some sense of support even in the midst of challenge and threat. My trust and faith might be a deep trust in my ability, as an expression of divinity, to be present with whatever arises. That is, I'm not trusting that this circumstance will turn out all right. Rather, I'm trusting that I can hold this circumstance in something wider and deeper, which is both beyond me and part of me, so that I can be with what is happening in this moment, even if it is not all right.

A second approach is to in some ways step out of the continuous search for safety and the illusion of control. This is not to say that we should not try to make ourselves and others as safe as possible; we should. Rather it is trying to recognize that no matter how safe we try to make ourselves and others, there is no way to achieve complete safety. Ultimately, we cannot control our experience. However safe we try to make ourselves, we could be hit by a bus, struck by lightning, or have a heart attack in the next moment. But still, we constantly tell ourselves, *If only X would happen* (I would get that job, get that person, have that baby, have those people like me, make more money, be successful), *then I would finally be truly safe, finally all right.*

When we recognize, however, that nothing we ever get or achieve, no fortress no matter how strong, will ever give us total safety, we can start to relax a little bit. Our desperation and rigidity can recede, because we see that they do not serve us, leaving a wise concern for our and others' well-being and prompting us to act in a reasonable and balanced way to protect ourselves and others. Once we accept, for example, that there is no way to be 100 percent safe from Covid-19 (or from losing our job), and that we do not have complete control, we can stop frantically obsessing about eliminating all possible risk and instead focus on taking smart precautions. Through both of these approaches, we can start to touch a basic *all-rightness* which is less dependent on how the world reacts to me or what happens in the world, but is rather more connected to something deep and essential within my being.

Conclusion

Building ourselves an ark through the practices we have explored can help us not only escape the flood, but perhaps even to delight in the vast waters which surround us—to see new possibilities and to release old ways of being. The Psalms tell us that the Leviathan, who swims in the "great and wide sea," the vastest of waters, was "created to play" (Psalms 104:25-26). What an extraordinary image. God creates the Leviathan for play. This is not the terror of Hobbes, but a vastness that invites our own majestic whimsy, creativity, and openness.

As we experience the terror, uncertainty, suffering, and loss of this plague, we can flood ourselves and get lost in the overwhelm. Or we can find presence, love, and beauty; discover support in the midst of fear; and unleash our creativity, responsiveness, and playfulness. This ark of wholeness can carry our joy *and* grief, our love *and* fear, our pleasure *and* pain. The invitation of the ark is to create buoyancy, vitality, love, and presence amidst what feels like an overwhelming flood—and so transform that flood into life-giving water. Afloat now on these waters, we can appreciate the sacred beauty of the vast ocean and sky which surround us.

Torah in a Time of Plague

History and Literature of Plague

Praying Away the Plague:
Jewish Prayer during the Italian Plague of 1630-1631[*]

Yitz Landes

It goes without saying that plague, and other forms of mass illness or death, present people and societies with myriad difficulties that manifest themselves on every plane of human existence and thought. In the realms of theology and religious practice, such calamitous circumstances raise questions like: What is the meaning of this catastrophe? How can theological and ritual frameworks provide space for so much death and mourning? How can prayer be most effective? And how should prayer even take place, given the risks and logistical difficulties imposed by plague?

In this essay, I will look at the ways North Italian Jews sought to pray— and to pray in a way they deemed most efficacious—over the course of the Great Italian Plague of 1630-1631.[1] The initial description will be based primarily on Abraham Catalano's *Olam Hafukh* ("The World Turned Upside Down"), a detailed account of the outbreak in the city of Padua. I will then turn to a cycle of prayers for plague found in Aaron Berechiah of Modena's 1624 prayer book *Seder Ashmoret ha-Boker*, as it is likely that Jews in various North Italian communities recited these prayers during the outbreak. Toward the end of the essay, I will look also at two briefer accounts of this outbreak, one in the autobiography of Leon Modena, a relative and contemporary of Aaron Berechiah of Modena who lived in Venice; and another in Avraham Masarini's chronicle, *Sefer ha-Galut veha-Pedut*, describing the outbreak in Mantua. As will be seen, a common thread in

---

[*] I had the opportunity to teach much of the following material on several occasions under the aegis of the Shalom Hartman Institute of North America; I would like to thank the Institute for providing me with these opportunities, and also the various participants in these classes for their comments. I would also like to thank Menachem Butler, Alyssa Cady, Susan Einbinder, Merle Eisenberg, Daphna Ezrachi, Yakov Z. Mayer, Shai Secunda, and the editors of this volume for their help in preparing this essay, particularly as my access to libraries has been significantly limited during this time.

[1] For the etiology of the North Italian plague of 1630-1, remembered as the worst outbreak in North Italy since the Black Death, see Alfonsina D'Amato et al., "Of Mice and Men: Traces of Life in the Death Registries of the 1630 Plague in Milano," Journal of Proteomics, Proteomics in Infectious Diseases, 180 (2018):128–37. On literary responses to this outbreak by Jewish authors, see Susan L. Einbinder, "Poetry, Prose and Pestilence: Joseph Cincio and Jewish Responses to the 1630 Italian Plague," in *Shirat Dvora: Essays in Honor of Professor Dvora Bregman*, ed. Haviva Yishai (Beer Sheva: Ben-Gurion University, 2019), 73–101.

these depictions and prayers is that disease is a result of sin; many prayers are thus penitential in nature. Other prayers hearken back to Temple rituals that were deemed efficacious in warding off illness.

The theological challenges that these Jews faced and their liturgical responses are both reminiscent of and in dialogue with the experiences of Jews during other epidemics. While it is wrong to assume that all diseases have the same impact and elicit the same responses, it is the case that a Jewish liturgical tradition surrounding outbreaks of disease does in fact exist. Thus, while my focus here is on one specific region and period, I believe that the texts I analyze here can shed light on the ways in which Jews have reacted to mass illness over the course of history and even in our own time.

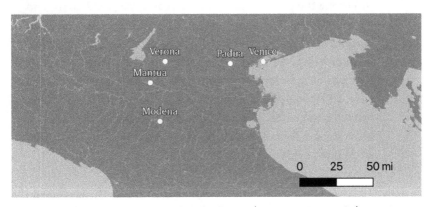

Map of North Italian cities mentioned in this chapter (Courtesy: Yitz Landes)

Abraham Catalano (d. 1641) was a doctor and rabbi who oversaw much of the medical response in the Paduan Ghetto during the outbreak of 1630-1.[2] *Olam Hafukh*, which he wrote in a beautiful, elevated Hebrew, is his attempt to summarize what he witnessed and experienced.[3] At the out-

---

[2] On Abraham Catalano, see David Malkiel, *Stones Speak: Hebrew Tombstones from Padua, 1529-1862,* Studies in Jewish History and Culture 43 (Leiden and Boston: Brill, 2013), 70-1, 301, who points out that Catalano's extensive epitaph speaks to his role as a doctor during the 1630-1 plague ("Of his having raised and sustained—sparing no pain—the one who bears His image and likeness, remind the Master with one voice").

[3] First published as Abraham Catalano, "'*Olam Hafukh*': The History of the Plague in the City of Padova" (Hebrew), ed. Cecil Roth, Kobez Al Jad IV (XIV) (1946): 65–102, primarily on the basis of London, Jews College, MS Montefiore 473. All translations from this work are my own, and are based on an earlier manuscript that Roth was unaware of, now New York, Columbia University, MS X893 Ab8. A partial translation of this work can be found in Alan D. Crown, "The World Overturned: The Plague Diary of Abraham Catalano," Midstream 19, no. 2 (1973): 85–76.

set of the work, Catalano states that his main reasons for writing *Olam Hafukh* are so that people will recognize God's strength and know how to properly prepare themselves, both as communities and as individuals, in the event of a future outbreak.[4] As he reports over the course of *Olam Hafukh*, Catalano's own household suffered immensely from the outbreak of 1630-1: Catalano's wife and four of his six children died in the plague. A son, Moshe, survived by taking refuge in Corte, and a daughter, Perla, survived in Padua.[5]

One of the first preparations taken by the Jewish community in Padua is immediately relevant to the topic of this essay:

> In Verona the plague started in the year 5390 [1629-1630] and we agreed here [in Padua] to entreat our brother, the *Aluf*, our Honorable Teacher and Rabbi, Solomon Marini, May God protect him—he found among his books a lengthy prayer that was written long ago in the city of Pisa, a large city of the wise, and it was pleasant in his eyes and he went, this *Aluf*, and printed it in Venice. And it was decided to recite it every week on Monday and Thursday after the Torah reading; and also, *Pittum ha-Ketoret*, every day, once the plague commenced.[6]

Once the outbreak had hit the nearby city of Verona, the leaders of the Jewish community in Padua realized that it may soon reach them as well. For Catalano and other leaders of the Paduan Jewish community, this meant that they would need to immediately prepare a proper liturgical

---

[4] *Olam Hafukh*, 73.

[5] The epitaphs of the Jews in Padua from the years 1529-1862 are well documented and have been collected and edited in David Malkiel, *Poems in Marble: Inscriptions from the Jewish Cemeteries of Padua, 1529-1862* (Jerusalem: Yad Izhak Ben-Zvi Press and The Hebrew University of Jerusalem, 2013), with further discussion in idem, *Stones Speak*. Yet Malkiel (*Stones Speak*, 338) notes that only one epitaph in this corpus—that of Malkah Lustro, who died on May 29, 1631 (*Poems in Marble*, 120)—records death by the plague of 1630-1, as the majority of the corpses were interred in an older cemetery outside the city gates that had long been abandoned; indeed, Catalano writes (*Olam Hafukh*, 84): "until the 16th of Sivan (=June 16th, 1631) the undertakers would take the dead to be buried in the cemetery in the city; but from the complaints of the nearby Sisters to the Judge they forbade us from burying here, and so we took them to the old cemeteries outside of the city." Catalano (*Olam Hafukh*, 82) mentions Malkah Lustro's death, and, as noted by Roth (fn. 6), her epitaph was written by Leon Modena (see Simon Bernstein, ed., *The Divan of Leo Modena* [Hebrew; Philadelphia: The Jewish Publication Society of America, 1932], no. 270, 251).

[6] *Olam Hafukh*, 73-4.

response. Calling upon Solomon Marini (d. 1670), the leading Paduan rabbi,[7] the community printed, in the neighboring city of a Venice, a liturgy to be recited during the outbreak, under the title *Tefila li-Zman she-Lo Tavo ha-Magefa* ("A Prayer for the Time of Plague, which Should not Come").[8]

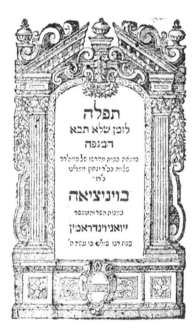

Tefila li-Zman she-Lo Tavo ha-Magefa (Venice: Vendramin, 1630)
Photo Courtesy of the National Library of Israel

This liturgy is still found today in a number of libraries.[9] Its central mechanism is one that is well known from many other genres of Jewish liturgy: in the absence of sacrifice to atone for our sins, it is hoped that reciting the details of the sacrifice will suffice. What is immediately striking, both from Catalano's description and from the prayer pamphlet itself,

---

[7] On Solomon Marini, one of the few Paduan rabbis to survive the outbreak, see Malkiel, *Stones Speak*, 307; and Hananel Nepi and Mordechai Shmuel Ghirondi, *The Memory of the Righteous for a Blessing and The History of the Greats of Israel and the Giants of Italy* (Hebrew; Trieste: Marenigh, 1853), 334, 336, 338.

[8] *Tefila li-zman she-Lo Tavo Ha-Magefa, asher nimtzeit bi-veit midrasho shel kevod moreinu ha-rav Shlomo ben rabbi Yitzchak Me-Marini* (Venice: Vendramin, 1630).

[9] For the purposes of this chapter, I used the scans of the copy found in the National Library of Israel, available online at https://www.nli.org.il/he/books/NNL_ALEPH001728155/NLI (accessed 8/5/2020).

is that the entire liturgy leads up to the recitation of the ingredients of the incense offering as they are listed in the Babylonian Talmud (b. Karetot 6a)—a prayer known as *Pittum ha-Ketoret*. The primary place given to the incense offering hearkens back to the Book of Numbers, in which it is said that Aaron used the incense offering to halt the plague outbreak that followed Korah's rebellion (Numbers 17:11-13). The connection between incense and plague is made in multiple points in the Zohar,[10] as well as in various other kabbalistic works, including ones composed in North Italy during this period.[11] It is important to recognize the ubiquity of *Pittum ha-Ketoret* in the context of protection against plagues, even in the absence of outbreaks. Marini's liturgy is only one example of many such usages of the *Pittum ha-Ketoret* in the history of Jewish liturgy; similar liturgical pamphlets based on the *Pittum ha-Ketoret* prayer have been printed many times in subsequent centuries—as recently, even, as during the Covid-19 pandemic.[12]

In addition to *Pittum ha-Ketoret*, Catalano mentions also the use of other well-known Jewish prayers, writing that "on the 11th of Sivan [5391, or June 11, 1631], we organized, the rabbis, that we should say in our prayers, in the evening and morning, the *Viduy* and *Al Heit* and *Avinu Malkeinu*, so as to stimulate heavenly compassion."[13] These three confessionary prayers are well known in the history of Jewish liturgy as prayers for forgiveness, to be recited on fast days and during the period leading up to the High Holidays.

It is apparent from Catalano's chronicle that most Jews no longer felt that it was safe to go to synagogue once the plague had reached the city. Catalano and other leaders of the Jewish community sought to ensure that some form of communal prayer would take place:

> And then we decreed on all unmarried men to come and pray
> outside of the synagogue of the Ashkenazim in the courtyard
> of the synagogue; and the Italians, in the women's section;

---

[10] See *Zohar*, (*va-Yakhel*), 2:218b.

[11] See especially Aaron Berechiah of Modena, *Ma'avar Yabbok* (Mantua: Judah Samuel di Perugia, 1626), 120b-121a.

[12] For one contemporary example, see *Kuntres Tefilot Meyuhadot li-Miniyat Mageifat ha-Corona* (Jerusalem: Nehar Shalom, 2020). In a forthcoming article, Susan Einbinder discusses the history of this prayer in the context of both Kabbalah and medical history; see Susan Einbinder, "Prayer and Plague: Jewish Plague Liturgy from Medieval and Early Modern Italy," in *Death and Disease*, ed. Lori Jones and Nukhet Varlik, (York: York Medieval Press, forthcoming). I would like to thank Prof. Einbinder for sharing this article with me prior to its publication.

[13] *Olam Hafukh*, 83.

so that there would be space between those praying. And we commanded that they pray early in the morning, before the heat of day, even on the Sabbath.[14]

For the Jewish leaders, it was imperative—for the community's sake—that able-bodied emissaries would pray together on behalf of the community. They thus specifically *ordered* the likely reluctant unmarried men to do so, as their illness or even death would not be as devastating as the death of an adult man with dependents. In order to do so somewhat safely, the communal leaders made sure that prayers would take place in the courtyard of the Ashkenazi synagogue and in the relatively spacious and ventilated women's section of the Italian synagogue, so as to maintain some physical distancing. And they ordered them to pray early, before the heat of day, as they thought the disease spread more easily in the heat.

Yet, as the outbreak took an even greater toll, even this did not work. Catalano writes:

> In those days, we were not careful in the rites of mourning... And the priests were not at all careful about the rules of impurity, as they did not want to move from place to place and reside in their fellow man's home, lest they contract the plague. And also, they would even take the dead for burial on the Sabbath, lest the fumes of their corpses lead to more death. And we also saw then that those coming to pray in the synagogue were few. And as the days progressed and the pestilence worsened and the number of stricken grew, they did not reach a *minyan*, to the point that we stopped praying in the synagogue for many days, and the "Small Temple" was desolate, without anyone visitors. And at times they would gather, with much exertion, in the synagogue of the Ashkenazim, and they would pray without keeping the normal order and tradition.[15]

Catalano describes a situation in which the plague and fear of death led to an almost complete abandonment of ritual norms; the main priority was avoiding the deceased and the diseased, to the point that the Sabbath was violated, the priests no longer maintained their elevated state of purity, and

---

[14] *Olam Hafukh*, 78.
[15] Ibid, 85.

the synagogue was empty. Communal prayer then only took place intermittently, and it was impossible to do so properly, since they could not gather a quorum of men who all prayed according to the same rite.

An exception, in terms of prayer practice, seems to have occurred in the month of Tammuz 5391 (July 1631). Catalano writes that this month was particularly difficult: "In those days, the voice of the Ghetto was heard—a wailing cry of bitterness, men and women lamenting The Tammuz, day and night—it would not stop."[16] Catalano's daughter Hana died on the 2nd of the month; his wife, Sarah, died on the 14th of the month; and two of his sons, Yehudah and Leon, died on the 25th. In the late afternoon of the Fast of the 17th of Tammuz, Marini ordered that all should clean the Ghetto, and then, following the afternoon prayers, he "took out two Torah scrolls and stood and prayed with the survivors in the Ghetto, on its four quarters,[17] and blew the shofar."[18]

* * *

Alongside the liturgical texts and practices described by Catalano, there is another set of prayers for plagues that was likely used during the North Italian outbreak of 1630-1. Beginning in the final decades of the 16th century, many Jewish men in North Italy began to form confraternities that would meet to pray in the early hours of the morning, prior to the daily morning prayer, known collectively as the *"Shomrim la-Boker"* ("Morning Sentinels") societies.[19] These groups eventually began to print small prayer books of the specific liturgy used by their confraternity, bringing together ancient and medieval prayers with prayers written by contemporary liturgists. As scholars have shown, these groups were inspired by the contemporary practices

---

[16] Ibid., 91; "בימים ההם קול הגיטו נשמע נהי בכי תמרורים אנשים ונשים מבכות את התמוז יום ולילה לא ישבות."

[17] Catalano earlier described that the Ghetto had been divided, for the purposes of the administration of health services, into four quarters.

[18] Ibid., 90; see also Mishnah tr. Ta'anit, 3:4. Catalano (91) writes that Marini also sought to institute an additional fast on the New Moon, to the consternation of his community, given the difficulty of the situation and the unprecedented nature of holding a fast on the New Moon festival.

[19] For a recent survey of these groups, their practices, and liturgies, see Michela Andreatta, "The Printing of Devotion in Seventeenth-Centuy Italy: Prayer Books Printed for the Shomrim La-Boker Confraternities," in *The Hebrew Book in Early Modern Italy*, ed. Joseph R. Hacker and Adam Shear, Jewish Culture and Contexts (Philadelphia: University of Pennsylvania Press, 2011), 156–70, 291-99.

of Safedian Kabbalists, who sought to hasten the redemption through early morning prayer.[20] Michela Andreatta has further argued that these groups were influenced by wider religious trends in Counter-Reformation Italy.[21]

In Modena, one such confraternity went by the name of *"Me'irei Shahar"*—"Those Who Awaken the Dawn," playing off both the time of day and the hoped-for hastening of the redemption.[22] Aaron Berechiah of Modena (d. 1639)—most famous for his extremely influential book on rituals surrounding death, *Ma'avar Yabbok* (Mantua 1628)—compiled this group's prayer book, printed under the title *Seder Ashmoret ha-Boker* in Mantua in 1624. Following a lengthy introduction and prayers for each weekday, for the Sabbath, the New Moon, Holidays, and Fasts, the prayer book includes cycles for calamities such as drought, torrential rain, epidemics, and the death of an important individual. The prayer book then moves to additional prayers for lifecycle events, and concludes with further remarks from Aaron Berechiah.

For our purposes here, the cycle for epidemics, entitled, *"Seder al ha-Holim,"* "Order for the Sick," is of course the most relevant. This cycle is built of three *selihot*—penitential poems—and two chapters of Psalms, as follows: (1) Psalm 38; (2) the *seliha "Eileha Adonai Nasani Eineinu"*; (3) the *seliha "Al Zot Te'eval ha-Aretz"*; (4) Psalm 41; and finally, (5) the *seliha "Avlah Navlah Tama ki-Shahar Nishqafa."*[23] This exact cycle of *selihot*, without the chapters of Psalms, appears in many medieval manuscripts of the Italian rite as prayers to be recited in the case of *"Ribui Holim,"* "[When] Many [have fallen] Ill."[24] It is important to note that this cycle, in both its manuscript and printed forms, was not copied or printed for a *specific* outbreak; rather, outbreaks of the plague or other epidemics were just one of the various calamities, natural or otherwise, that one could expect to occur with some frequency and that one needed to prepare for liturgically.

The earliest of the three *selihot* in the cycle for mass illness is most likely the middle one, *"Al Zot Te'eval ha-Aretz,"* and it was composed by the late 9th to early 10th century South Italian liturgical poet Amitai b. Shefatia.

---

[20] See already Moses A. Shulvass, *Rome and Jerusalem* (Hebrew; Jerusalem: Mosad HaRav Kook, 1944), 110-14.

[21] Andreatta, "The Printing of Devotion."

[22] Ibid., 293.

[23] Aaron Berechiah of Modena, *Seder Ashmoret ha-Boker* (Mantua: Judah Samuel di Perugia), 206a-209a.

[24] See, for example, Parma, Biblioteca Palatina, MS 2403 (De Rossi 963; Richler 903), 405v-407v—an early 14th century Italian Mahzor.

Amitai's *seliha* is representative of the themes found in many of the *selihot* for outbreaks of illness, both in this cycle and in other rites:

על זאת תאבל הארץ,׳
כי אין איש גודר פרץ,
ואין משליך מידו השרץ,
לכן מתגרים תחלואים בכליון וחרץ:

אמנם אנחנו פשענו ומרינו,
כי מדת אבותינו בידינו.
נא מדתך לא תשנה בעבורינו,
ורפואתך מהרה תקדמנו:

מאז זאת לעולם נצבת,
בעשות תשובה בת שובבת.
מדת רחמים לא מתעכבת,
כי יד דוחה וימין מקרבת:

תחלואים ונגעים ופגעים,
ראויים למענגים ומשעשעים,
ולא לעם עייפים ויגעים,
אשר ימיהם מעט ורעים:

יום יום מחכים לתשועה,
והנה לאות ויגיעה,
בין מצד גזירה רעה,
ובין במכה המהלכת בכל שעה:

יה אם הרבינו חובות,
וקץ הגיע שטר לגבות,
בתשות כחנו השקיפה מערבות,
כי בידך למעט ולהרבות:

חיתנו בידך פיקדון מקימת,
בין להחיות ולהמת.
חלילה נאם תרעומת,
כי אנחנו הרשענו ואתה עשית האמת:

יהמו רחמיך וחסדיך,
על עם עבדיך ועדיך,
לצוות למשחית מפי כבודך,
'רב עתה הרף ידיך':

העלה ארוכה ותרופה,
על אום חולה דוויה וסגופה,
כי לך זועקת ומצפה,
'ובעמך לא למגפה':[25]

"For this the Earth shall mourn" [Jer. 4:28],
As no person can close the breach,
And nobody releases the varmint from their hand,
The ill are thus confronted with death and destruction.

Although we have sinned and disobeyed,
We hold yet our ancestors' merit in our hands,
Please, do not change Your manner with us,
And may You quickly bring forth Your healing.

From the beginning it stands,
A way for the rebellious daughter to repent;
Your measure of mercy, do not withhold,
For the left hand pushes away and the right brings close.

Illness, pestilence, and affliction
Befit the comfortable and the amused,
But not a nation that is tired and weary,
Whose days are short and bitter.

Day by day they await salvation,
Filled with weariness and fatigue,
Whether from the evil decree,
Or from the blow that strikes at every hour.

---

[25] The text here is based on that in Parma MS 2403, 405v-406r (and differs slightly from the text printed in Yonah David, *The Poems of Amittay: Critical Edition with Introduction and Commentary* (Hebrew; Jerusalem: Achshav, 1975), 62-64; the English translation is my own.

Lord, if we have amassed debt,
And the time has come to collect the bond,
Look, from heaven, upon the tired ones,
For it is in Your hand to reduce or to increase.

Our lives, in Your hands, are a secure deposit,
Whether to live or to die.
Heaven forbid, a disquisition of rage!
For we have sinned, and You did what is right.

May Your compassion and kindness spring forth,
Onto the nation of Your servants and witnesses,
Command the affliction, from Your honorable mouth,
"It is enough, stay thy hand!" [2 Sam 24:16].

Raise up a cure and a medicine,
For the nation that is sick, sad, and suffering,
For to You it cries out and looks,
"And let not Your people be plagued" [1 Chron. 21:17].

The *seliha* consists of nine stanzas, and is built on a central theme common to all *selihot*: our present suffering is due to our sins (both communal and individual), and we pray that God forgive us. The sins here are unspecified, but the unwillingness on the part of the community to change their ways is likened in the first stanza to individuals who try to purify themselves in a *mikveh* while holding a rodent or bug that voids their purification process.[26] Those praying beseech God to focus not on their sins, but on the merit of their ancestors, and to allow them to repent—a process, it is recalled, that God set in place even before He created the world.[27] In the fourth and fifth stanzas, Amitai notes that the People of Israel are particularly unable to confront the epidemic: they are "tired and weary" from their general suffering, as they sustain blows from both the disease and "the evil

---

[26] For this imagery, see already Tosefta tr. Ta'aniyot 1:8 (Lieberman ed., 326).

[27] See Genesis Rabbah, 1:4 (Theodor-Albeck ed., 6); the use of the Hebrew word "מאז" in this line plays off the way in which this midrash reads the pre-Creation period of time signified by the word "מאז" in the verse "יי קנני ראשית דרכו קדם מפעליו מאז" (Prov. 8:22, "The LORD created me at the beginning of His course, as the first of His works of old"), which is read as the Torah's self-description as having been created prior to creation.

decree"—that is, from the anti-Jewish policies of their non-Jewish rulers. They entreat God to forgive their debt, and then, in the *seliha's* climax, they acknowledge that this request is somewhat arrogant—"For we have sinned, and You did what is right."

Over the course of the final two stanzas, the *seliha's* request is framed in simple terms—"May Your compassion and kindness spring forth… Raise up a cure and a medicine…" These two stanzas incorporate biblical passages in which God halts outbreaks of mass illness. The first of these quotations is of God's direct speech to an angel of affliction, in which, before the angel reaches Jerusalem, God tells them, "It is enough, stay thy hand!" (2 Sam 24:16). This imagery plays off the earlier references to hands in the *seliha*: the people of Israel do not release the creepy thing from their hand when they attempt to purify themselves in the *mikveh*; God's left hand pushes away but his right hand brings near; it is in God's hand to reduce the punishment; and then, finally, God tells the plague itself to put down its hand.[28]

Amitai's *seliha* is written, like all *selihot*, as a particularistic prayer for the Jewish people. As such, it is also framed as a *communal* prayer—it comes from the lips of the Jewish people, as they pray to God on their own behalf. As is common in liturgical poetry, Amitai left his individual stamp on the composition by signing his name in an acrostic: thus, the first letters of the second to fifth stanzas spell out the name *"Amitai."* Yet the signature continues in the following stanzas, leading to a full acrostic of *"Amitai Yihye"*—"Amitai Shall Live." In this way, the liturgical poet also inserts his own personal prayer into the *seliha*, asking that *he* should survive the outbreak, and he also reflects on his ability to continue to live on through his literary composition.

Returning to the North Italian outbreak of 1630-1, it is quite probable that many Jews would have recited this *seliha*, along with the other two that appear in Aaron Berechiah Modena's *Seder Ashmoret ha-Boker*.[29] Yet, they would have mostly encountered Amitai's *seliha* with a few significant differences. In the version in *Ashmoret ha-Boker*, the entire fourth stanza is missing, and in the fifth stanza, the line "Whether from the evil decree" was replaced with the phrase "major misfortune," such that the stanza reads

---

[28] I would like to thank Rabbi Naomi Levy for calling my attention to the importance of the hand imagery in this seliha.

[29] On the extent of the 1630-1 plague outbreak in Modena, see Mirko Traversari et al., "The Plague of 1630 in Modena (Italy) through the Study of Parish Registers," Medicina Historica 3, no. 3 (2019): 139–48 (who note that the outbreak began there already in 1629).

Day by day they await salvation,
Filled with weariness and fatigue,
From the major misfortune—
The blow that strikes at every hour.[30]

These omissions and changes are due to the censoring of Hebrew books on the part of the Christian Inquisition. The fourth stanza, in which the *seliha* describes the People of Israel as being particularly unready to withstand an outbreak of mass illness would have been interpreted as a prayer that the disease should instead afflict the non-Jewish population (dubbed "the comfortable and the amused"). Relatedly, either the censor (or, fear of the censor) would have prevented the direct reference to Christian imposition on the Jews. Indeed, the spread of disease was at times thought by Christians to have been the fault of the Jews. Some Jewish authors even describe the anti-Jewish tension that arose when outbreaks first took root in Christian quarters and only belatedly seeped into the somewhat-isolated Jewish neighborhoods; Catalano claims that the plague only reached the Paduan Ghetto months after the initial outbreak in the city, and that Jews thus "feared the non-Jews" of the city, as "their jealousy was raging."[31]

***

As a doctor, rabbinic figure, and writer, Abraham Catalano bore witness to the deaths of hundreds of members of his community. He ends the narrative of the events a beaten man. The last paragraphs of *Olam Hafukh* list suggestions for how to prepare in the event of a future outbreak, and the majority have to do with forms of social distancing, either by locking oneself in a room or, ideally, retreating to the countryside. He then appended a series of short poems by his surviving son, Moshe, that contain

---

[30] Modena, *Seder Ashmoret ha-Boker*, 207b.

[31] *Olam Hafukh*, 77. Catalano writes earlier (73) that Christians feared that Jews would bring the plague to Padua, on account of their cross-regional trade; meanwhile, he writes (78) that many Jews believed that the plague reached the Ghetto via the family of the Ghetto's non-Jewish gatekeeper (73). In addition to what Catalano describes in *Olam Hafukh*, see also the similar situation in the Venetian Ghettos as described in Leon Modena, *The Autobiography of a Seventeenth-Century Venetian Rabbi: Leon Modena's Life of Judah*, trans. Mark R. Cohen (Princeton: Princeton University Press, 1988), 135-36; for Mantua, see Einbinder, "Poetry, Prose and Pestilence," 80; and more generally on the delayed infestation of the Ghettos, ibid., 99. See also the depiction of the outbreak of the plague in Rome 1656-7 in Jacob Zahalon, *Otzar Ha-Hayyim* (Venice: Vendramin, 1683), 21a.

similar messages.[32]

Leon Modena of Venice (d. 1648), Catalano's contemporary and Aaron Berechiah's cousin, ends his less detailed depiction of the outbreak in Venice on a slightly different note[33]:

> As mentioned before, the plague continued in the city and among the Jews through Heshvan 5392 [November 1631]. Then God in His great mercy took pity, and the bitterness of death turned away. There was great celebration in the city, and everyone gave thanks to his God. In addition, a fast was decreed in all the holy congregations for the eve of the new moon of Kislev, with a prayer service for the new moon during the day, including *"Nishmat Kol Hai"* and with the pleasant sound of joyfulness. A collection was taken up in every synagogue, which will be used to make a silver object to commemorate the deliverance. *Blessed is He who redeems and saves, blessed is He and blessed is His name.*[34]

According to Leon Modena, to mark the end of the outbreak, the day before Rosh Hodesh Heshvan 5392 (October 23, 1631) was marked as a fast for the entire community.[35] In addition, the New Moon festival itself was celebrated with additional, festive prayers, and the community financed silver objects to donate to the synagogues in order "to commemorate the deliverance." Similarly, Avraham Masarini writes that the Jews of Mantua "all went to the Great Synagogue and recited the extended *Hallel*" when a

---

[32] On these poems and for a translation of the first of them, see Einbinder, "Poetry, Prose and Pestilence," 78-80.

[33] On the impact of this outbreak on the population of Venice, see the Adelman and Ravid's notes in Modena, *The Autobiography of a Seventeenth-Century Venetian Rabbi*, 244-46, who note the existence of a mass grave in the cemetery that served the Venetian Jewish community that has the simple marker "1631 HEBREI" (see also Adelman's comments in his introduction on pages 32 and 40).

[34] Modena, *The Autobiography of a Seventeenth-Century Venetian Rabbi*, 137. For the original Hebrew, see Leon Modena, *Chayye' Yehuda: The Autobiography of a Venetian Rabbi*, ed. Daniel Carpi (Hebrew; Tel-Aviv: Tel-Aviv University Press, 1985), 86.

[35] At the time, some Jews in North Italy had recently taken up the custom of observing the day before the New Moon as a fast day, which is referred to as a *Yom Kippur Kattan*, "A Minor Yom Kippur"; see Elliott Horowitz, "Jewish Confraternities in Seventeenth-Century Verona: A Study in the Social History of Piety (Italy)," (PhD dissertation, Yale University, 1982), 99-102. It is notable that Modena does not make an explicit connection here in his autobiography with the practice of Yom Kippur Kattan, yet it is certainly possible that this practice influenced the decision to fast on the day before the New Moon.

wave of this epidemic ended on the 6th of Av of 1630 (July 15, 1630), a year or so before it would end elsewhere.[36] These practices are echoed in yet other Jewish accounts of outbreaks of plague,[37] as well as in the contemporary Christian practice.[38]

* * *

We have seen here that during the North Italian plague outbreak of 1630-1, the leaders of the Jewish communities in the affected cities understood that a liturgical response was needed—one that was based on specific liturgical texts appropriate for such a situation. These prayers were not necessarily "new," but were framed as old, potent prayers that needed to be printed and distributed quickly. Two of the prevalent forms of prayer were the recitation of the *Pittum ha-Ketoret*, the ingredients of the incense offering, deemed particularly effective at warding off plagues; and the *seliha*, a common genre of penitential prayers in which the devout seek forgiveness for their sins. In addition to finding appropriate prayers, leaders of the Jewish communities sought also to ensure that prayer would take place, and in as responsible a fashion as possible. And lastly, they chose to mark the end of the outbreak liturgically and with donations to the synagogues.

The texts analyzed here present an understanding of plague as having come about primarily due to sin. Effective prayers would thus petition God for atonement, either through direct confession or through the nostalgic reframing of ritual mechanisms deemed to have been effective in the utopic, Temple-centric Jewish past. Indeed, for the authors of these texts, plague is just another feature of the Exile, as the Jewish people continue to suffer "Whether from the evil decree / Or from the blow that strikes at every hour."

---

[36] Avraham Masarini, *Sefer ha-Galut veha-Pedut* (Venice, 1634), 12a.

[37] For a slightly later example see, Zahalon, *Otzar ha-Hayyim*, 21b.

[38] See Adelman and Ravid's notes and references in Modena, *The Autobiography of a Seventeenth-Century Venetian Rabbi*, 246.

Torah in Troubled Times:
Experiencing Epidemic in Prague, 1713

Joshua Teplitsky

Torah occupies a privileged place in Jewish tradition as a sustainer of life, even, in some texts, as life itself. Jewish prayers assimilate verses from Proverbs and elsewhere to cast Torah as "a tree of life for those who cling to it" (Proverbs 3:18). What happens, however, when death—in the forms of plague and pestilence—strikes? How are the institutions, individuals, and legal traditions bound up with Torah study and Torah law affected by plague? And how, most importantly, do the dictates of Torah and tradition interact with human exigency, experience, and emotion during a time of crisis, fear, and pain? While no single source, book, or experience can stand in for the whole, a micro-historical approach—one that combines sources from law, literature, and liturgy to reconstruct the particular experiences of individuals in time and place—offers a unique vantage point to examine up close the impact of plague on the rhythms of Torah study, halakhic decision-making, and ritual practice as manifest in real human life. To appreciate the impact of epidemic on daily life, culture, and community, we'll peer into the world of one man who was touched by epidemic—and follow his thought and experiences.

Our guide will be a man named Jacob Reischer (c. 1660-1733). A Prague native, Reischer (sometimes also referred to by the surname Back or Backhoffen) lived and served as a rabbi and judge in a number of Jewish communities in Central Europe, including Worms (in western Germany) and Metz (in eastern France), as well as in Prague and parts of Bohemia (today's Czech Republic). A fierce intellectual and author of several books, Reischer could be a contentious figure. His positions were sometimes so controversial that his colleagues wrote entire treatises disagreeing with his stances.[1] Reischer's experiences and writings grant us a singular vantage point from which to examine epidemic in Jewish history and its effect on Torah and law in everyday life.

Reischer was no stranger to plague. It struck his native Prague once in 1680 and a second time in 1713, claiming approximately a third of the

---

[1] Shmuel Shilo, "Ha-rav Ya'akov Raischer ba'al ha-sefer Shevut Ya'akov: Ha-ish bi-zemano li-zemano veli-zemanenu?" *Asufot* 11 (1998), 65-86.

population on each occasion. Bubonic plague (also called the Black Death), caused by the bacterium *Yersinia pestis*, was a part of early modern life—a period historians of disease refer to as the "Second Pandemic" which extended from the first outbreak of the Black Death in 1348 to the receding of the plague from Europe after 1720.[2] The Bible, Talmud, and other Jewish writings from antiquity through the Middle Ages all feature episodes of epidemic. But the period after 1348—with the introduction of plague as a nearly-endemic condition of early modern life—was a time when plague featured prominently in a wide array of writings by and about Jews. Virtually every surviving memoir written by Jews during this period recounts the experience of living through plague. Some Jewish writers tell of the family they lost to disease, such as the Venetian rabbi Leone Modena.[3] Others, like the female memoirist Glikl of Hameln, relay the panic and confusion that even a suspicion of plague could provoke. One year during Sukkot there was concern that her daughter might have contracted the plague; the Jews of her community fled the synagogue and drove the family into hiding from the neighboring gentiles.[4] An anonymous Hebrew autobiographer from seventeenth-century Bohemia (the modern Czech Republic), relays the precarious situation Jews faced between the limited protection of rulers and the danger of popular hostility.

That anonymous autobiography also tells us something about the intimate experiences of Reischer and his household during a plague outbreak in 1680:

> In 5440 (1680) a plague broke out in Bohemia, and especially in Prague. From that city the Rabbi, R. Jacob Backoffen (Reischer), the author of Minhat Jakob, came with his wife Jettel and her sister Freidel, the daughters of the Rabbi, R. Wolf ben Rabbi Simon Spira [the chief rabbi of Prague and Bohemia]; and they stayed with us in our house in the village. I still remember the great modesty of that scholar who was willing to take the trouble

[2] I. Bos et al., "A Draft Genome of Yersinia Pestis from Victims of the Black Death," *Nature* (London) 478, no. 7370 (2011): 506-10. Lester K. Little, "Plague Historians in Lab Coats," *Past & Present* 213, no. 1 (2011): 267-90; Frank M. Snowden, *Epidemics and Society: From the Black Death to the Present* (New Haven, CT: Yale University Press, 2019), 40-42.

[3] Mark R. Cohen, *The Autobiography of a Seventeenth-Century Venetian Rabbi: Leon Modena's Life of Judah* (Princeton, NJ: Princeton University Press, 1988), 137.

[4] Chava Turniansky, *Glikl: Memoirs 1691-1719*, trans. Sara Friedman. (Waltham, MA: Brandeis University Press, 2019), 107-114.

to teach me like a school teacher.[5]

Reischer and his family's first recourse during plague was to flee. Such an approach was part of the conventional wisdom of Christians and Jews alike. A Hebrew medical manual of the period entitled *Be'er Mayyim Hayyim* (The Wellspring of Living Waters), conveyed the conventional wisdom that dated back to antiquity that the first remedy of the plague is "to run away...far, immediately, and for a long time."[6] Early modern people facing plague often left their homes and communities in dread and out of a sense of self-preservation that they might avert the worst by abandoning the affected place.

Often, however, the attempt to outrun the plague kept people from staying put anywhere for long, as they strove to outpace the pestilence. The autobiography continues:

> But his wife, who domineered over him, did not permit him to carry out his good intention. In the course of Tammuz I fell sick, and the symptoms of the plague became apparent. For three days and nights I had high fever and was near death. Then a swelling broke out behind my ear on the neck which burned like fire, and all the members of the family became frightened. The Rabbi and his wife noticed it, and fled from our house to the house of his uncle in Wotitz [Votice, a town about 40 miles from Prague].[7]

In the young author's telling, Reischer was cast as compassionate, while his wife's fear prevented his "good intention" and ultimately forced the family into further flight from the plague.

Reischer's wife's instincts, however domineering or alarmist they seemed to the young observer, may have saved his household. Yet flight from an

[5] Alexander Marx, "A Seventeenth-Century Autobiography: A Picture of Jewish Life in Bohemia and Moravia: From a Manuscript in the Jewish Theological Seminary," *Jewish Quarterly Review* 8 (1918): 279 (Hebrew); 293 (English).

[6] This was itself a quotation of the Latin dictum Issachar "primum remedium fugit." See Issachar Bär Teller, *Be'er Mayim Hayyim* (Prague, 1650). A translation is available as *The Wellspring of Living Water*, trans. Arthur Teller (New York: Tal Or Oth Publishers, 1988), 53. On the work, see Jean Baumgarten, "Un Livre De Médecine En Yiddish: Le 'Beer Mayim Hayyim' D'issachar Ber Teller (Prague, Seconde Moitié Du Xviie Siècle)," *Revue Des Etudes Juives* 168, no. 1-2 (2009) : 103-129.

[7] Marx, "A Seventeenth-Century Autobiography."

afflicted city was fraught with both practical and theoretical challenges. Intellectuals, both Jewish and Christian, debated the religious permissibility of fleeing from a city, raising important theological concerns about the significance of attempting to evade divine decrees. Some understood plague as divine intervention, a direct and unmediated act of God upon the world. This perception was given voice in the Bible itself. II Samuel tells us that when King David conducted a census of his subjects, God was angered with this action, and sent a prophet to offer the king his choice of punishment: a seven-year famine, military loss, or a three-day plague. David chooses the last option, saying "Let us fall into the hands of the Lord, for his compassion is great, and let me not fall into the hands of men" (II Sam. 24:14), demonstrating that while all three punishments came from the Divine, plague marked the most direct assault upon humans by God without intermediaries. For some Talmudic thinkers and later halakhists, flight from the city might represent a rejection of the divine plan and would be worthless as an attempt to escape fate, while others saw it as a lifesaving measure and a religious duty.[8]

In debating this matter, Jewish thinkers had much in common with their non-Jewish neighbors and contemporaries. Christian thinkers of the Middle Ages and early modern period debated the virtues, or vices, of flight as a response to plague. The reformer Martin Luther dedicated one of his writings to the question "On Whether One May Flee from a Deadly Plague" in 1527 and again in a 1542 tract entitled "Should ministers flee in times of pestilence?"[9] Notably, Luther remarked upon Jewish responses to plague in the course of his discussion, writing that "it pleases me very much that the Jews apply the psalm, 'He who dwells in the shadow of the Most High' [Ps. 91], to the pestilence," a psalm that explicitly mentions disease ("that He will save you from the fowler's trap, from the destructive plague").[10] Luther likely meant that Jews recited the psalm, either individually or in collective prayer, as a means to ward off illness; this psalm was often uttered

---

[8] Moshe Dovid Chechik, "Ha-Isur o he-hovah livro'ah min ha-ir be-sha'at ha-magefah," *Ha-Ma'ayan* 233 [60, 3] (2020): 22-34; Moshe Dovid Chechik and Tamara Morsel-Eisenberg, "Plague, Practice, and Prescriptive Text: Jewish Traditions on Fleeing Afflicted Cities in Early Modern Ashkenaz," *Journal of Law, Religion and State* 8, no. 2-3 (2020): 152-78.

[9] See Dean Philip Bell, "Ministry and Sacred Obligation: A Late Medieval Context for Luther's 'on Whether One May Flee from the Death'." In *The Medieval Luther*, ed. Christine Helmer (Tübingen: Mohr Siebeck, 2020), 197-212.

[10] *Luther's Works, vol. 54: Table Talk*, ed. and transl. Theodore G. Tappert (Saint Louis, MO: Concordia Publishing House; Philadelphia: Fortress Press, 1955), 119-38.

as part of the deathbed rituals of early modern Jews as well.[11]

Theoretical debates only captured part of the matter. As Reischer's case indicates, when confronted with the reality of plague, rabbis—like numerous others—took whatever measures they could to save themselves and their families, often taking flight themselves. Beyond the immediate personal implications for health and well-being, self-imposed exile in the face of plague also affected the professional output of rabbis and authors. Various early modern scholars recorded the impact on their process of composing new works of Jewish literature. Some lamented the impact of plague on their scholarly lives and harkened to such moments to account for lags in productivity or lacuna in their knowledge. Most famous among these is Rabbi Moses Isserles (the Rema, 1530-1572) who, during an epidemic in Krakow in 1556, took refuge in Zhidlov.[12] Others, however, saw in their refuge from plague an opportunity to think and write, unhindered by the norms of daily life and communal obligation. Hayyim b. Bezalel of Friedberg (1520-1588—the brother of the famed Maharal) contrasted the flight from yeshivas in 1569 and its concomitant disruption of study with his own persistence, as he endeavored to uphold his study routine, "a refuge from the angel of death," eventuating in his book *Iggeret ha-Tiyul*.[13] He credited another epidemic, of 1578—which claimed the life of his maidservant, threatened the life of his son, and kept him shut in for a period of nearly two months—with creating the conditions for him to write his *Sefer ha-Hayyim*.[14]

If for some fortunate individuals the act of flight offered escape from danger and even opportunity for creativity, for those left behind the results were demoralizing and chaotic. In the late summer of 1713, plague struck the city of Prague for the second time in Reischer's life. The outbreak disrupted manifold aspects of life in the city, disrupting market exchanges and daily encounters between Christians and Jews, halting movement in

---

[11] Jacob Rader Marcus, *Communal Sick-Care in the German Ghetto* (Cincinnati, OH: Hebrew Union College Press, 1947), 269.

[12] Moses Isserles, *Sefer mehir yayin* (Hamburg, 1711), 2r.

[13] Hayyim b. Bezalel, *Iggeret ha-Tiyul* (Offenbach, 1717; first published Prague 1605): introduction.

[14] Hayyim b. Bezalel, *Sefer ha-Hayyim* (Krakow, 1593): introduction. A number of other authors indicated their writing activities during times of plague, see Abraham Yaari, *Mehkerei sefer: perakim be-toledot ha-sefer ha-ivri* (Jerusalem: Mossad Harav Kook, 1958), 90-99, and more recently the sources collected in *Ne'emnu Me'od: Eduyot gedolei Yisrael al halikhoteihem u-minhageihem bi-yemei holi u-mageifah* (Jerusalem: Mekhon Yerushalayim, 2020), 170-176.

and out of the city, and claiming the lives of nearly a third of the city's inhabitants, Jewish and Christian alike. Plague also disrupted Torah study, both in affecting the operation of institutions and as an object of scholarly decision-making. A Yiddish poem printed shortly after the epidemic's conclusion captured the trauma to Torah institutions:

> May it never befall you, all who pass along the road [Lamentation 1:12], that which has happened to us. We have seen the departure of the sagely head of the rabbinical court and the yeshiva. The beauty and light of the entire Jewish community. Who will protect us now?

> From the four corners of the earth young men had come, and as they wanted to escape the plague, they left as soon as it began and returned home.

> Now the great Torah that is learned by us and which sustained us, we have so soon lost. In all the streets and houses one heard nothing but the Torah as it used to be studied.

> The elixir of life which is the reward of Torah study has escaped us; on account of our many sins death has begun instead.[15]

The poem registers the pain of those left behind, not only as they compared their unfortunate circumstances to the ones who fled, but also as they expressed anguish that Torah and its students, a sustaining element of Jewish community, had now been wrenched from them.

Epidemics affected more than the elite institutions or individuals engaged in Torah study; these plagues raised new questions about Jewish law, life, and ritual in ordinary life. Reischer's close encounters with plague—and his record for posterity of the questions he faced as a rabbi and judge—

---

[15] Moses ben Hayyim Eisenstadt, Eyn Nay Kloglid (Amsterdam, n.d.), 2v. For a variant translation see Sylvie-Anne Goldberg, *Crossing the Jabbok: Illness and Death in Ashkenazi Judaism in Sixteenth- through Nineteenth-Century Prague*, trans. Carol Cosman (Berkeley: University of California Press, 1996), 163-164. On Yiddish plague poems from Prague, see Chava Turniansky, "Yiddish Song as Historical Source Material: Plague in the Judenstadt of Prague in 1713," *Jewish History: Essays in Honour of Chimen Abramsky*, ed. Chimen Abramsky, Ada Rapoport-Albert, and Steven J. Zipperstein (London: P. Halban, 1988), 189–98.

allow us to see beyond the experiences of an individual and his family and into the lives of his contemporaries. His responsa (*She'elot u-teshuvot*) offer a glimpse into a variety of ways that plague affected Jewish life, and the ways that he and others attempted to accommodate and expand the domains of Torah to grapple with these dramatic events. The following three responsa reflect poignant moments from the epidemic of 1713, and offer insights into moments of hardship, anxiety, and legal dilemmas. They encompass issues of marriage, sex, and procreation; communal charity and relief; and burial.

Sex in a Time of Plague

In one responsum, Reischer records a question he received regarding sex and procreation during plague, as follows:

> In the year 1713 when there was a plague (*dever*) in Prague I was asked by a man, who was frightened and trembling that he had not yet fulfilled [the commandment to] be fruitful and multiply accordingly, if it was permissible to serve the bed or not, as is noted in the glosses to the Shulhan Arukh in O[rah] H[ayyim] item 240, sub-sign 12, citation "with other misfortunes such as hunger," these are the words of the questioner.[16]

Surrounded by illness and death in the present, the questioner contemplated bringing life into the future. There is perhaps no greater investment in the future than bringing children into the world, yet what could be more frightening than the prospect of bringing vulnerable innocents into danger? The question begs for balance between pausing the normal rhythms of life in the midst of crisis and anticipating normalcy in times to come. It also may be motivated by the questioner's fear of his own mortality—the worry that he himself may perish in the plague without having fulfilled his earthly duties, thus compromising his immortal soul.

In responding to the question, Reischer drew upon an array of sources to thread a delicate needle that offered autonomy for the decisor and the questioner alike. He did this by distinguishing between different degrees of childlessness, noting the difference between literal childlessness and the rabbinic understanding that a man (the subject of the religious requirement to procreate) does not technically fulfill his obligation until having children

---

[16]Jacob b. Josef Reischer, *She'elot ve-teshuvot shvut Ya'akov*, 3 vols. (Metz, 1789), 3: no. 30.

of both sexes. Whereas in ordinary times a man would be expected to father at minimum a child of each sex, a more literal definition allowed leeway in establishing the degree of one's obligation to procreate even during a crisis, and forgave the "trembling" questioner from worry that he had not done his duty.

Reischer's line of reasoning allowed that even fathering a single child would suffice to fulfill this man's obligation. But he was also sensitive to the fact that this man may have *wanted* to father more children, and therefore veered away from warning him off of it entirely. Reischer concluded his responsum by ruling that abstinence was a mark of piety, but was not obligatory. He wrote, "since it is only the measure of piety it is permitted."[17]

Notably, Reischer grounded this opinion not only in his questioner's possible desire to have children, but also in an acknowledgement of the power of human sexual desire, even when the world is turned upside down. He continued, "since there are grounds to be concerned that if he does not serve [the bed, i.e., if he does not have procreative sex] he shall come to sin, either he or his wife if she yearns for him."[18] Reischer's analysis moved beyond a question of simply whether one should have children into an acknowledgement of sexual desire and its power to move people to act. Although he framed this concern in terms of avoidance of sin—either through fears of adultery or even wasted seed—his acknowledgment of sexual desire as an overriding factor recognized it as deep, intrinsic, and motivating, and a force to be reckoned with, not denied or ignored. Just as importantly, Reischer acknowledged desire's presence in partners of both sexes, and noted that such desires needed satisfaction through legitimate channels, lest the partners seek outlets elsewhere. As such he validated sexual desire even during a time of crisis.

Social Support in a Time of Plague

If plague could disrupt the most intimate of family situations, it also had consequences for the public realm as well. The onset of plague was not solely a matter for deliberation over individual choices, but also affected the community and its energies during a time of scarcity and panic. Plagues and pandemics disrupt not only the rhythms of daily life but bring markets and economies to a grinding halt, robbing individuals and families of income.

[17] Reischer, 3: no. 30.
[18] Reischer, 3: no. 30.

Still worse, epidemics also disrupt the mechanics of charity, welfare, and the organized distribution of resources that might ameliorate poverty and neediness. In Prague's 1713 outbreak of plague, as Jews and their communal institutions struggled to meet the needs of the ill and indigent, Reischer grappled with the following query regarding diverting resources from other sources to poverty relief:

> Question: A terminal patient who instructed before his death that a certain sum of his money should be used for the ransom of captives, and now that the noise of plague is in the world, may it be kept from us, in the year 1713, and many of Israel are in dire straits, if it is permissible to give them [i.e., those in dire straits] this money or if it is a deviation from the intention of the donor.[19]

The question reflected the difficult economic circumstances wrought by epidemic, and the abiding desire to respect the will of donors. Reischer was at great pains to approve of the repurposing of these funds during an epidemic; the Talmud (Bava Batra 8a) had established captivity as the most severe of fates, more punishing than famine or the sword, and had therefore reserved funds for the ransom of captives.[20] And yet Reischer argued that the talmudic hierarchy was not entirely apt for his own time. Reischer suggested that the world was different in his time than in former times, when "the hand of God was in the world" and Israel "acted with kindness one to the other."[21] As in the responsum treating procreation, famine stood in for plague as a biblical reference point for total catastrophe and lack.

Reischer argued, instead, that the outbreak of an epidemic resulted in a form of captivity on par with literal imprisonment:

> But now, on account of our sins, the burden of exile has multiplied upon us, and the false libels of our enemies who libel against us that the plague comes on account of Israel. And when there was plague in the year 1713 in many places in

---

[19] Jacob ben Josef Reischer, She'elot ve-teshuvot shvut Ya'akov, 3 vols. (Halle, 1719), 2: no. 84.

[20] On the ransom of captives in early modern Jewish life, see Adam Teller, Rescue the Surviving Souls: The Great Jewish Refugee Crisis of the Seventeenth Century (Princeton, NJ: Princeton University Press, 2020), especially 116-123. On the dynamics of early modern Jewish charity and communal control see Debra Kaplan, The Patrons and Their Poor: Jewish Community and Public Charity in Early Modern Germany (Philadelphia: University of Pennsylvania Press, 2020).

[21] Jacob ben Josef Reischer, She'elot ve-teshuvot shvut Ya'akov, 3 vols. (Halle, 1719), 2: no. 84.

which there were members of our people they had closed the Jewish street with literally none coming and none leaving, and at great pains by intercession they were allowed to bring them necessary alimentation, and in some places they had to go and hide themselves in forests and caves, and [people of] Israel that were on the road and in the fields were abandoned to die... there is no greater captivity than this...[22]

In this responsum Reischer unleashed the full force of his personal anguish over the plague in Prague of 1713. He noted obliquely that Jews were deemed responsible for plague, which resulted in the closure of their neighborhood. Indeed, when the plague broke out in the summer of 1713, medical experts and governing authorities singled out Prague's Jewish quarter for special attention and segregation out of fear that it was a hotspot of contagion. Jews in Prague had lived in a bustling but cramped neighborhood that by the early 18th century had numbered over 11,000 Jews in a relatively small area known as "the Jewish Town." Christian travelers to Prague during the 17th and 18th centuries repeatedly remarked upon the overcrowding of this ghetto, noting the unsanitary conditions that prevailed within it. Jews also belonged to a highly mobile sector of the local population, with students, merchants, and the vagrant poor entering and exiting the city. One medical expert identified the Jewish Town as a vector in the spread of the disease on account of Jewish fur traders who had recently arrived in the area from Poland, where the plague had hit earlier in the year.[23] Reischer thus confidently ruled that repurposing funds from the ransom of captives to the support of those besieged by plague and by government discrimination was by no means a deviation from the will of the donor, as "there is no greater captivity than this," identifying quarantine itself as a prison and a captivity.[24]

Burial in a Time of Plague

Reischer was not wrong that the authorities had attempted to segregate Jews, and in so doing had imprisoned them within the walls of their own

---

[22] Reischer, 2: no. 84.
[23] Alexander Anton Ignaz Schamsky, *Freund in der Noth, oder kurtzer und grundlicher Unterricht, wie Jeder bey jetzt grassirenden Seuchen sein eigener Medicus seyn solle* (Prague, 1713), 1–2.
[24] Reischer, 2: no. 84.

neighborhood. Instructions from even the earliest moments of the plague called for separation, washing, and instructions for burial. The state of medical science of this period understood the transmission of disease less in terms of contagion and more as a result of environmental factors, and believed that the foul air from decomposing bodies could pose a significant threat as a source of plague itself. The same Yiddish poem that described the denuding of the Prague ghetto of Torah and its students (quoted above) also relayed the material impoverishment of the Jewish community and the hardships surrounding burial, noting that:

> When someone would die, he could not be buried in the cemetery of the street [i.e., the Jewish cemetery in the center of the Prague Jewish Town], rather he had to be taken, led, or carried to the *lazaretto* [plague hospital]. Who could look upon the misery and pain?[25]

Burial of bodies was done partly by wagon and also by sending bodies downstream to a newer cemetery than that which lay at the heart of the Jewish quarter. But burial instructions were more detailed than just location. The government mandated swift burial, deep in the ground, and stipulated that the body be covered with quicklime before covering it with earth.[26] These instructions prompted a new question for Reischer.

> Question: At the time of the plague, may it be kept from us, in the year 1713 when the sovereign, his highness, instructed in one of the places that one was not to bury the dead in the cemetery of their fathers that is in the city without first pouring lime upon it to decompose, and if not, to bury him in one of the forests in which there is no human settlement, which is preferable?[27]

The questioner offered a dilemma between obeying the new sanitation orders, which might violate the integrity of the deceased body, so valued by Jewish burial law, or burying in a remote location, potentially consign-

---

[25] Eisenstadt, *Eyn Nay Kloglid* (Amsterdam), 4r.
[26] Národní Archiv (National Archives Czech Republic), Prague, Ms. Stará manipulace 842/E2/16, box no. 663: folio 4r.
[27] Reischer, 2: no. 97.

ing the dead body to be lost to future commemoration. The discussion revolved around the use of quicklime, a chemical agent that prevents putrefaction. This was crucial to early modern medical thinking, which understood plague as transmitted through miasma in the air as a product of rotten remains.

Reischer drew upon medieval discussions of the Rashba (Solomon ibn Aderet, 1235-1310, responsum #369), who discussed exhuming bodies and the religious permissibility of adding decomposing agents (perhaps understanding the power of quicklime not as preventing decomposition but avoiding putrefaction). Rashba's discussion weighed concerns that altering the decomposition of a dead body might be a degradation and dishonor to the body and might, moreover, cause the body (or the departed soul of the body) pain. Although Reischer acknowledged the indignity of such an act, he concluded that "in our case it is preferable to pour lime upon him and to be buried in the burial neighborhood, and not to bury him in the forests like the burial of a donkey, without guardianship, for it is possible that there the dogs will dig him up and carry him off, and the like. It appears simple to me."[28]

Reischer once again weighed the present against the future, balancing dignity and exigency. His instructions about burial and the importance of placement in the cemetery bore additional significance as cemeteries were not solely sites for the dead, but for the ritual life of the living as well.[29] The particular importance of plague commemoration in the cemetery persists in a small pamphlet printed in Prague in 1718/9, some five years after the plague had abated. The pamphlet comprised a Yiddish prayer, or *tkhine*, entitled "A new *tkhine* for the people who died in the plague." This prayer belonged to a genre of Ashkenazic women's spirituality and ritual activity of the early modern period called *tkhines*. The most famous of these, *The Three Gates* by Sara bas Tovim, relayed a centuries-old custom of measuring the cemetery or individual tombstones with candlewick, and then preparing candles during the High Holiday season, usually burning them on Yom Kippur.[30]

---

[28] Ibid.

[29] On the cemetery as a space for both the dead and the living in Prague, see Rachel L. Greenblatt, *To Tell Their Children: Jewish Communal Memory in Early Modern Prague* (Stanford, CT: Stanford University Press, 2014), 47-82.

[30] Chava Weissler, *Voices of the Matriarchs: Listening to the Prayers of Early Modern Jewish Women* (Boston, MA: Beacon Press, 1998); Yemima Hovav, *'Alamot Ahevukha: Hayye Ha-Dat Veha-Ruah Shel Nashim Ba-Hevrah Ha-Ashkenazit Be-Reshit Ha-'Et Ha-Hadashah* (Jerusalem:

This "new *tkhine* for the people who died in the plague" may well have been designed to accord with this custom. In this slim publication, the reader of the prayer was directed to ask God for forgiveness for her inability to properly identify the graves of the lost, to commemorate the anniversary of death with precision, and, moreover, for her failure to weave a burial shroud for the unknown deceased and the array of other last rites that they deserved. The text referenced elements of the Yom Kippur prayers, especially the harrowing *Unetaneh Tokef,* which proclaims acceptance of the divine judgement even as the reader begs forgiveness and intercession. The *tkhine* also invoked aspects of the Yom Kippur liturgy by referencing the Ten Martyrs at the time of the Temple's destruction, perhaps in the process invoking an understanding of the victims of plague as holy martyrs themselves.[31] The publication of this *tkhine* points toward the long period of reckoning that followed the outbreak of the plague in a way that complements Reischer's inclusion of his plague responsa within his wider oeuvre.

In time, life in the city of Prague returned to the normal rhythms of what had come before. A Jewish traveler to the city in 1719 recorded the hustle and bustle in the Jewish Town, noticing the fullness of its market, synagogue, and street life, as well as its remarkable cemetery.[32] Plague had receded, the absent voices a memory. Yet its impact remained in writings, in recollections, and in legal traditions and challenges bequeathed to posterity, recorded by Reischer and others in recognition that, having come in the past, plague could rear its head once more. Reischer was a man who thought

---

Merkaz Dinur, 2009). On rites in the cemetery of early modern Ashkenazic communities during the High Holiday season and their implications for communal and social hierarchy, see Debra Kaplan, "'The Poor of Your City Come First': Jewish Ritual and the Itinerant Poor in Early Modern Germany," in *Connecting Histories: Jews and Their Others in Early Modern Europe,* ed. Francesca Bregoli and David B. Ruderman (Philadelphia: University of Pennsylvania Press, 2019).

[31] Eliot Horowitz has noted the looming presence of martyrological thinking in early modern deathbed rituals, suggesting that the very need for a presence of a minyan (a prayer quorum of ten men), engendered a spiritualized martyrdom that saw in every death an opportunity to sanctify the divine name through a form of sacrifice. Elliott Horowitz, "The Jews of Europe and the Moment of Death in Medieval and Modern Times," *Judaism: A Quarterly Journal of Jewish Life and Thought* 44, no. 3 (1995): 278-279. On the power of martyrdom in early modern European Christianity, see Brad S. Gregory, *Salvation at Stake: Christian Martyrdom in Early Modern Europe,* Harvard Historical Studies (Cambridge, MA: Harvard University Press, 1999). See also Edward Fram and Verena Kasper-Marienberg, "Jewish Martyrdom without Persecution: The Murder of Gumpert May, Frankfurt Am Main, 1781," *AJS Review* 39, no. 2 (2015).

[32] Shlomo Berger, ed, *Travels among Jews and Gentiles: Abraham Levie's Travelogue Amsterdam 1764* (Leiden, Netherlands; Boston, MA: Brill, 2002), 69.

about plague and guided others, but his texts were not simply those of a man at remove. A survivor who fled earlier outbreaks of plague, Jacob Reischer was a man who directly confronted the 1713 plague both personally and professionally, and his works offer insights into the resultant disruption to Torah institutions, even as they testify to the flourishing of Torah thinking. Reischer's responsa, like other texts and sources from the period, bear witness to loss and recovery. In him we can see Torah during a time of plague as it was understood, as it was experienced in institutions, and as it struck deeply at the heart of Jewish daily and communal life. Both individual and collective commitments did not cease. Outbreaks of epidemic prodded new writing and thinking, and prompted halakhic creativity. Indeed, as scholars and lay people alike attempted to uphold their commitment to Torah's dictates and institutions, Torah was not only impacted by plague, but also served as a guide to weathering crisis and catastrophe, and to renewing life when plague subsided.

Quarantine Reflections

The Song of Sirens: A Covid Birth Story

Tamara Mann Tweel

I looked up at the fluorescent lights, the flimsy blue sheet separating me from my stomach, and tried to pray. I could hear sounds coming into the room: a nurse or a loudspeaker repeating "move all Covid patients to Floor 7." Was I on Floor 7? I scanned the walls. No, this must be Floor 2. What about the pre-op room where I just waited for two hours? Are they talking about me? My mind raced, fastened to a now familiar anxiety: did I wash my hands, were we far enough apart, did I have Covid? What about my baby? My baby. I came back to the room, I came back to my body. I pushed the unforgiving anxiety away. I prayed. I beseeched. Then the magnificent drama began. Not of fear and disease, but of the blessing of new life. Frenetic movements paused as the doctor lifted my baby up beyond the blue sheet. I heard my child cry. I lingered on his full head of silky dark hair. I noticed the speckled red dots on his nose. And I craved his scent. My newborn came to me, into my arms, onto my chest, and all was good.

On March 29th, at the height of the Covid-19 outbreak in New York City, my son's gentle cry cut into a room, into a hospital, into a city overcome by fear and grief. When I try to make sense of that moment, I fixate on the sounds. The tears of nurses as they struggled with securing protective equipment, the snaps of masks on and off, the Purell pumps, the feet shuffling to stay distant—and always, always, the sirens, transporting the ill from home to hospital, and the bodies from hospital to earth.

I kept my newborn son, all seven pounds of him, in the crook of my arm, as nurses ushered my husband out of the hospital. I was moved around and around, back to the pre-op room, into an elevator, onto a hallway, and finally onto what they called the "Covid-free floor." The nurses looked tired; the janitor looked scared. Finally, we came to our resting place, near a window, and it was evening.

I heard my roommate turn, the soft blue shade between us rustle, as she slowly moved left and right in her cot. My body seized with panic until I felt the baby, soft and sweet, gently breathing on my chest. What time was it? The banging outside the window grew louder. I could hear the confident voice of a foreman, or was I imagining the sound? It must have been 2:00 or 3:00 a.m., but I felt enveloped in a construction site. I breathed with my newborn child. I felt peaceful in my sea of white mesh gauze and eagerly eyed the tray at my left, which housed a prized carton of whole milk my roommate had secured for me. Three days in, she was an old-timer, an arrival from Jackson Heights, Queens, who had labored alone and delivered a baby girl. I heard the girl whimper and her mother pick her up. "Do you hear that noise outside," she asked me. "I'm glad I'm not hallucinating. What do you think is happening?" My roommate rose, opened the window, and we watched as the park across the street from our hospital room transformed into a giant tent city, an outdoor hospital across from a hospital, awaiting what our nurses called "the surge."

While enraptured by new life, we were both surrounded by the threat of death. Mothers have been here before—in war, in famine, and in childbirth—we knew. But our past experiences had ill prepared us for desert tents awaiting urban trauma. I inhaled and brought in the sweet-smelling scent of my newborn child. I called my husband and my two older children and shifted uncomfortably as the full reality of my wounded body took hold. I remember well the pain. The pain was almost a relief, the externalization of a kind of spiritual discomfort I had been enduring for months. The alluring strangeness of this miraculous birth had begun earlier, in a different era, when our personal, and not global, struggles still carried weight.

Ten months ago, I turned 40. Nine months ago, I found out I was pregnant. After a decade of pregnancies, two miraculous children and two second-trimester miscarriages, I had thought the years where I would expand and contract were behind me. And yet, in my late thirties, I began to feel an indentation in my chest, a kind of spiritual desire that physically hollowed me. I would dream of this little soul whispering near me, asking to be born. I believed that the act of creating life was a religious affirmation, the strongest way to live the truth that God knows more than we do; that the future is more important than the present; that life itself is more precious and more holy than our vision can ever truly grasp. And so we tried for another child, although I assumed it would never happen. Pregnancy had never come easy to me.

The reality of this late-in-life pregnancy astonished me. Rather than a feeling of purpose or joy, I was overwhelmed with panic. How would I do this? How would we afford our lives? What would I tell my new employer? The petty logistics of my crass materialism overtook me and I felt deeply unworthy. I felt unworthy of this miracle. Rather than being filled with holiness, I was filled with logistics, with small crises, with inherited worries that had somehow become my own. Late at night, as I heaved into my pillow, my husband looked at me, concerned: *Isn't this what you wanted, what you prayed for? This is good. Just wait darling. Just wait.*

My dear friend came to my home to pray with me, but I felt far from God. My failure to experience the blessing of this pregnancy haunted my religious life. I stopped going to shul. I said it was the pregnancy, but it was more than that. I stopped learning Torah. I said it was work, but it was more than that.

As I grew far from my faith, my husband grew closer to his. My husband converted to Judaism almost 15 years ago. He fell in love with our rituals at home, with learning Torah, and with the deep friendships we formed over long Shabbat meals. He had always been a full participant in our religious life, but while he was my partner, I was often our family's conduit to Judaism. In this pregnancy, my husband became our family's spiritual anchor. He learned Rambam once a week with a rabbi and dear friend; he studied the prophets; and left for shul early with our son, beaming when our 6-year-old put his kippah on and sat next to him to pray. I lived in a spiritual home, even though I was filled with spiritual doubt. I was grateful for that. I was also grateful for the habits of faith that kept me rooted: Shabbat, religious school for my children, my monthly Torah group, and my cousins. But beneath the habits was an ache. A sense of purpose lost, of mission diluted, and of faith unmoored. This was in November, December, January and February. This was before March.

Busyness can be a spiritual salve. Life fills up. The blessed bounce of urban chaos occupied my days as I jumped between work and children. I woke up to the hustle of school lunches, drop-offs, recycling, commutes, emails, and finished the day with bedtime routines, dirty dishes, and more emails. I lived beholden to my calendar, constantly trying to move this around to make that. My two-bedroom apartment was crowded, one husband and two children, but crowded in a way that felt alive. In those early spring days, we were preparing as a family to welcome our third child. On March 7th, I was working on the menu for the bris. And then the waves of realization came, in stages, crumbling the fortress of movement, halting my sense of time and belief in a stable future. The spiritual ache turned physical.

First my husband, a physician in New York City, came home from a day of emergency room call concerned. His medical practice would temporarily close. He would be furloughed. And then my children came home. Their school would close. The fear began to set in. The fear of economic insecurity, the fear of death, the fear of having the last precious years of childhood seized. Joan Didion has a line in her novel *Blue Nights* about this kind of loss: "The fear is not for what is lost. What is lost is already in the wall. What is lost is already behind the locked doors. The fear is for what is still to be lost."

My early moments of stress were naive. The deaths hadn't come yet. As March wore on and my skin stretched to accommodate new life, I began to hear of the losses—a friend's mother, a past colleague, 5,000, 10,000, 20,000 dead. The city filled up with the endless sounds of sirens. And the pain, jobs lost, savings destroyed, loved ones without protective equipment serving on the front lines. Beyond the ongoing anxiety I felt for my children, for my husband, for my parents, and for my city, was an almost constant spiritual cramp, the doubt about bringing new life into this very dangerous and insecure world.

When Odysseus faced the prospect of the Sirens, he asked to be tied to the mast of his ship. He knew the sounds would entice him to abandon his mission, toward chaos, and toward death. My sirens would not beguile me with beauty, but they would invade me with thoughts of anxiety, mortality, and agony. What would I use to insulate myself? On March 25th it looked like I would deliver this child alone. Spouses were forbidden from entering the hospital. I reached out to my teachers, asking them to send me texts— from the Torah, from literature—to bind me, to protect me, to elevate me, as I waited to deliver.

On March 28th, Governor Andrew Cuomo intervened and demanded that all hospitals in New York allow partners for the delivery but not the rest of the hospital stay. And so at 5:00 a.m. on March 29th, my husband and I arrived at the hospital with a folder of texts from my teachers. We started the day with blood tests, nose swabs, IV lines, and Melville, with Ishmael's reflection on the sight of mother whales nursing in *Moby Dick*: "But far beneath this wondrous world upon the surface, another and still stranger world met our eyes as we gazed over the side. For, suspended in those watery vaults, floated the forms of the nursing mothers of the whales..." There was more to the quote but we couldn't get past the phrase "watery vaults." It is where we longed to be, somewhere enclosed and thick and peaceful. And so we conjured that underwater lake that Melville described and tried to steal ourselves into ourselves and away from the clanks and screams, vomiting and tears, that filled the small ill-designed room of thin-cloth separators and square tiled ceilings, where pregnant and newly nursing mothers waited.

When my husband left and my baby slept upon me that first day, his silk-velvet skin emanating with warmth, I unfolded the other texts. I read the texts bestowed upon me by rabbis and Jewish scholars, religious mentors, and friends. My body seized with discomfort at the distance I had created, the distance between myself and my faith, between my texts and my life. This is the Torah that found me in the pandemic; the texts my mentors and friends chose, as ropes upon the mast, to elevate and protect me in a time of great personal need.

Our dear friend, one of the rabbis who had nourished our home by learning with my husband, offered Pesachim 116a in the Talmud and asked why we dip *maror* into *haroset*? Why isn't it sufficient to just experience the bitterness? Reading the text again, through our friend's interpretive moves, transported me to that feeling I once had of yearning for the soul now breathing in my hands. Our friend explained that there have always been and will always be moments of sweetness and hope that emerge from bitter times. This is a truth and not a dismissal of pain. Optimism in dire conditions, he explained, is brave. It inspires humanity to create and build and endure. He cited Rashi on the connection between *haroset* made of apples and the orchards where the Jewish slaves of Egypt gave birth. When you dip the bitter herb in the thick *haroset*, the bitterness is consumed by hope. That is the gift of new life. It is always the gift of new life, in any and all conditions, but especially in times of great pain and of growing cynicism.

I let the shame wash over me. The shame that lived within me for nine months, the shame of being unworthy of this child. The shame of being fearful of economic uncertainty and change. The great shame of allowing myself to move away from rather than close to God. I looked at my newborn, so fragile and so sturdy, divine and human, his eyes watery vaults, his life a sign of redemption in chaos. His life an all-consuming hope.

When I entered the hospital, I planned to leave before we chose a name. I wanted to be with my husband and children and choose a name together that hewed closely to the experience of witnessing our son. After twelve hours in a hospital responding, as best it could, to the pandemic, I decided to leave early to heal at home with my family. At fifteen hours I was told that it would be almost impossible to name the child after I left and that it would be best to fill out the paperwork now. The ongoing dance between logistics and grandeur startled me. I would choose a name now, not because I was ready but because the bureaucratic paperwork required I do so. And outside—the sirens, persistent and piercing, moving the sick and dead.

I picked up another text, this one from my beloved childhood teacher, who helped me build a faithful life as a teenager. She brought me to the previous week's Torah portion and the building of the *Mishkan*. She wrote about Bezalel, the man tasked with leading the project of building a dwelling place for God on earth and the particular form of wisdom God gives to the builders of the *Mishkan*, "*chochmat lev*," or wisdom of the heart. While one might expect wisdom to be associated with the head or the brain, in this moment of sacred building, it is associated with the heart. As I pondered this trait of *chochmat lev*, I thought back to my own classroom, where I spent many summers teaching Socratic wisdom, a form of wisdom centered on the limits of human knowledge. Intelligence of the mind can be steeped in a dangerous form of surety. But wisdom of the heart is centered on true humility. It is this form of humility that gives one strength to bring holiness into this world. I thought back to my husband, who told me humbly to "wait," who offered me patience and faith amidst uncertainty. I looked down at my son, I repeated the story of building the *Mishkan*, a wandering home in the desert, I repeated the story of his father, and I called him Bezalel.

How does Avram become Avraham, began another note from a friend. It begins when Avram encounters a *birah doleket*, a glowing palace. He faces a place that does not make sense, a place that is simultaneously creation and destruction, order and chaos, beauty and pain. Drawing on Genesis Rabbah 39:1, my friend explained, we expand, we grow, we increase in holiness—when we endure the true visceral paradox of mortal existence. I took his words in. I looked outside my window and watched as holy men and holy women labored, moving cots and medical equipment, boxes of N-95 masks, and water bottles. I looked inside my room, at the careful way the nurses had prepared gauze strips and diapers. I listened as I heard them shuffle between rooms, healing despite their fear. I looked at my son, peaceful in my arms. I looked at my body, scarred and sore. And I listened to the sirens. The sick were coming. I let all of it in, the *birah doleket*, the palace and the flame.

Before I left the hospital, I gave my son his English name: Raphael.

In the twilight hours, between reading, nursing, listening, and witnessing, I fell in love with my son. I fell in love with the speckles on his nose, the curls forming by his ears, the way the bones of his chest breathed into my hands. I fell in love with his eyes. I became enclosed in his goodness and holiness. In Genesis 18, when Abraham exhibits his signature virtue of *hachnasat orchim*, hospitality, he is visited by three angels. In the Rabbinic tradition, it is claimed that one of these three angels is Raphael, who comes as a messenger of God, to heal Abraham. Raphael is a conjunction of two words, Rapha and El, meaning that God heals. As I prepared to leave Mount Sinai carrying a vision of the *Mishkan*, I came to believe that my dear child was an expression of this name. An expression not of surety and not of simplicity, but of the possibility that we can all be vehicles of divine restoration.

When Raphael was born, my life before him ceased to exist. With a new life came a new world. I am humbled by it all. My pain, my challenges, our agony, our losses have not been resolved. But Torah again flows into my life. God looks up at me from the watery vaults, and another sound pierces through the glissando sirens, thick and sonorous and round, *tekiah gedolah*, and together, Raphael and I are awake.

(Tractate) Shabbat in Quarantine

Ethan J. Leib

Daf yomi ("a page a day") is the world's biggest book club. Participants read a full folio of Talmud every day for seven-and-a-half years while staying on the same page as Jews around the world. I got notice that my day job was going remote, and that my kids were going to be home indefinitely, on the day Tractate Shabbat began in the *daf yomi* cycle. The previous tractate, Berakhot—or blessings—ended on March 7, 2020. With blessings feeling like they were coming to an end too soon, it seemed clear that my lockdown would at least be accompanied by a brand new book that might carry me through. The book takes 156 days to complete. And although my *siyyum* (a traditional party reserved for finishing one of these books) for Tractate Berakhot had to be cancelled because gatherings of friends were off-limits, I could try to look forward to August 10, 2020, when I could perhaps see my *havruta* (learning partners) again to celebrate the completion of Tractate Shabbat. That wasn't ultimately to happen, in light of where the pandemic took us all: even after we all cautiously emerged from our caves, much like Shimon bar Yochai, we had to go back in all over again (Tractate Shabbat 33b). That extended period of isolation permitted me to learn an extraordinary amount in those 156 days—and it turned out that learning with my *havruta* online meant I didn't have to keep entering a synagogue (which I had to for the previous tractate). It was a relief, really, to migrate *daf yomi* away from the shul and into Zoom: going to shul and putting on my kippah each week was alienating because unlike the rest of my *havruta* group, I wasn't interested in going upstairs to pray after our discussions of the week's pages.

This essay explores resonant themes in Tractate Shabbat for managing pause—and focuses some attention on the regularity of companionship *daf yomi* can provide even when we are otherwise alone and out of time. The tractate covers the laws surrounding the day once a week—the Sabbath—that Jews commit to going on lockdown, even when there is no plague around them. Although I do not observe Shabbat, Tractate Shabbat allowed me to observe it up close at just a time when everything around everyone was no longer following the pace of days and weeks and months and weekends and holidays that usually break up the calendar. Jews are serious about their calendars, of course, but one could be forgiven for thinking that almost all of those 156 days felt like a *bein ha'shemashot*—neither here nor there, a kind of twilight (the standard translation), neither day nor night, a signifier of sorts for the evanescent temporary and temporally indeterminate. These particular 156 days of *bein ha'shemashot* felt nothing like Rabbi Yosi's sense of the period as the "blink of an eye" (Tractate Shabbat 34b). Tractate Shabbat itself seems uncertain about what to say about this "period of uncertainty" (Tractate Shabbat 34a). Discussions of this netherworld of neither coming nor going appear dozens of different times in the book—more than any other book in the Babylonian Talmud—without clear resolution about its status. The most romantic description is Rabbi Hanina's claim about Rabbi Nechemiah's measurement of its duration: "When you can still see the top of Mount Carmel at the seashore, descend and immerse yourself in the sea and emerge—that is Rabbi Nechemiah's measure" (Tractate Shabbat 35a). The waters for me were too cold in Lake Russell with the Berkshires in the backdrop to make any effort to approximate *bein ha'shemashot* in real time.

* * *

In Ilana Kurshan's memoir about her own experience with a prior *daf yomi* cycle, she writes that "part of the experience of learning the Daf Yomi cycle is the dissonance between the subject of the tractate under study and the period it coincides with in the Jewish calendar."[1] She has in mind something like the reality that Passover 2020 started on the evening of April 8, during lockdown, but those in the current *daf yomi* cycle wouldn't get to the tractate that principally covers the laws of Passover until November 23. To be fair, though, that tractate would eventually conclude March 22, 2021—and five days later we'd have another seder.

Still, there were definitely some strange moments during the 156 days, when the pages covered just about what was going on in the Jewish calendar: The festival of Shavuot was May 28 to May 30 in 2020—and the only pages in all of the Talmud that cover that holiday were studied May 31 to June 2 (Tractate Shabbat 86b-88a). The nine days that lead up to the fast of Tisha b'Av that commemorates the destruction of the Temple

---

[1] Ilana Kurshan, *If All the Seas Were Ink: A Memoir* (New York: Picador, 2017), 272.

Torah in a Time of Plague

started on the day of Tractate Shabbat 138, which begins a recounting of prophecies about the ways Torah will be forgotten by the nation of Israel and the ways that Jerusalem will be destroyed. The page one learned in the lead-up to the ninth day of the month of Av (Tractate Shabbat 145) did not quite quote from the Book of Lamentations (the book that Jews read aloud on the ninth, which admittedly appears on 25b and 118a), but there was an overt reference to dirges from Jeremiah 9:9. Dirges—*kinot*—are traditionally read on Tisha b'Av after the Book of Lamentations. Jeremiah 9:10 explicitly envisions Jerusalem turning into rubble and into a den for jackals, an image redolent of what Jews would read in Lamentations 5:18 that evening in which the author laments that Mount Zion is desolate and "jackals prowl over it."

Quite apart from the *daf* cycle's contemporaneity with the Jewish calendar in these small ways was a deeper sense that Tractate Shabbat was speaking—if not on every page, in every chapter in some way or other—to the contemporary moment of pausing. Near the middle of the book, we are made to understand that the Sabbath—the day of pause—is not really just Saturday, the shorthand Jews use all over the world. Rather, it is a time that can be anytime, even when you lose all track of what day it is in the real world. Since all the days tended to bleed into one another during lockdown, Tractate Shabbat 69b was there to help orient and reorder those who were wandering in the wilderness. To be sure, the rabbis debated whether to observe a special day when you notice you are lost and then to count six (Chiya bar Rav) or instead to count six days and then take a special day—whatever day it happens to be (Rav Huna). What mattered more to me than how to resolve the rabbinic dispute was the reminder that no matter how lunatic and off-kilter the dissipation of time itself felt, there was always a reminder from 69b that people themselves could reclaim control of which day was which. And the book was telling you how to do it, too: by wearing special clothes (or maybe just putting on actual pants!) (113-114); by picking a day not to run (113); by altering your mode of thinking (113, 150); by not reading ordinary things (which in this time probably meant taking a day off from reading obsessively about the pandemic) (149a).

Tractate Shabbat wasn't only meditating on time and how to mark it just when time was warping; it was also improbably somehow talking directly to more practical worldly things going on around us. The very first page of the book (2a) tells a story about a poor person standing outside and a homeowner standing inside, figuring out how to send items in and out of the private and public domains, a central problem for Jews on Shabbat. The issue of how to carry and move things from one domain to the other occupies almost a third of the book. This spoke directly, it seemed, to many people's public health and moral dilemmas of the moment: whether to use Instacart shoppers; whether to interact with them at the door; how to keep our families guarded inside ethically when we know so many cannot afford to lock themselves in; how long to leave groceries untouched before allowing them to come in from the public domain to the private domain. The very fixation on domains, so central to Tractate Shabbat, spoke to how we think of our private spaces (even if we had abandoned our homes in hot spots), just when they were getting so much more private and the public domain was becoming ever more distant. Even when you crossed the threshold into a place that would once have been part of the public sphere, you were still bringing the privacy of the home outdoors with you. A discourse on whether you can even open a window on Shabbat (125b-126b) not only explicitly raised questions about the permanence of structures (and just how permanent quarantine was going to be was always in question), but also invited constant reevaluation of boundaries, as people started wondering who they were willing to welcome into their domains and where.

Then there were just eerie ways the Talmud was talking to those living in the time of the pandemic. For example, the most prominent measurement that appears in the tractate—about 120 times—is "four cubits." Consider 96b: "The Gemara holds that it is clear that parties kept their distance from each other. If they were nearer than the four cubits, they would reach each other with their needles and spikes and hurt one another." Four cubits today is translated as about six feet, the most religious of measurements to help us avoid the spikes of the novel coronavirus.

Or consider what seems like a mystery outside of pandemic times: Why does Tractate Shabbat derive so many of its rulings about the pause and quarantine of the Sabbath—about what is permitted and prohibited—from the rules surrounding laws of purity and impurity (e.g., 59a, 60a, 63a-64a, 66a, 112b)? Even the rabbis are sometimes puzzled by what the rules of impurity have to do with Shabbat: "Abaye asked: Are we really so simply learning the laws of Shabbat from the laws of impurity?" (123a). The link felt pervasive but tenuous—until one fully inhabits the pause and quarantine brought on by the pandemic. That entire experience was suffused with the worry about corrosion, contagion, and cleanliness, making the Shabbat-impurity link seem obvious. Learning what was and wasn't permitted during pause had everything to do with how corroded things were in the midst of the Covid-19 pandemic. Hand sanitizer and Lysol worked as the proverbial red heifer and ritual bath, even as Tractate Shabbat reminds us on 108b and 109a not to have our hands touch any part of our faces and to wash our hands three times to get the evil off them.

On 62b, the Talmud reports Rav Chisda's pronouncement that washing his hands well was the key to his well-being and success. This seemed like much better advice than the long list of incantations and folk remedies the rabbis recommended for dealing with fevers of various durations and intensities, like "dust from seven door sockets," "seven cumin seeds," and "seven hairs from the beard of an old dog" (66b-67a). There was something there for other symptoms, too, like what sounded similar to Covid toes (though may have been for random boils and wounds) and "demons of the bathroom" (67a). But the handwashing advice seemed like the right one to be heeding.

It was also hard not to hear in one's gut Rav Hamnuna's view on 119b that a nation was destroyed when schoolchildren were not able to study together in school. As the quarantine lingered in the United States, it seemed increasingly likely that face-to-face school was not going to be a full-time endeavor for the next academic term. Parents trying to work with kids around all the time did seem like the recipe for the destruction of a nation Rav Hamnuna was warning about. Maybe the thing to do was right there on 127a: "Once upon a time Rabbi Yehuda HaNasi [the spiritual leader in Tannaitic times who is credited with compiling the Mishnah] appeared at a place and saw that it was too crowded for students. So he found a field and cleared it in its entirety [to make room for all the students]."

* * *

One of the central prohibitions on the Sabbath is objects in the category of *nolad*: those items that were given birth as some kind of new creation or vessel on the very day when you are supposed to be on pause (Tractate Shabbat 28b-29a, 45b, 124b). The idea that pause should really be a time to do nothing, to not create anything new, made sense in the days of being cut off.

As it applied to the pause of the pandemic, there was a deeper lesson that was underscored by the artist Jenny Odell, author of the timely *How To Do*

Nothing.[2] Odell suggested that it was important for her to resist the urge to make something new and create art during quarantine. I heard her as saying—though I can't remember exactly what she said at double speed on the Vox podcast of the day—that the art of quarantine was almost surely likely to end up trite in part because of the universality of the experience, something that might take away from the singularity of the artist's voice. She highlighted that resonance in art—when the work feels right and familiar and recognizable—is part of what makes it successful. But she warned that if is it too familiar, there is a risk that the perceiver of the work too much thinks their experiences are either being exploited or that they could have done the work on their own, triggering dismissal, jealousy, or resistance. A challenge of creating in a pause that always feels immediate and looming is sustaining at least some kind of distance, necessary to make something truly artful.

Although *daf yomi* isn't exactly taking on Odell's challenge of "doing nothing"—every day of quarantine I probably spent more time learning the *daf* than any other single thing other than sleeping—I had early on tried to commit to doing it only *lishmah*, for its own sake, not to create from it. My career as a legal academic might be enhanced by learning this wellspring of Jewish law, but I write in other fields and wanted to "do the *daf*" as some kind of pause from all the other reading and writing about law I otherwise do all the time. Odell's warning notwithstanding, however, I couldn't help taking notes for a paper about pause and Shabbat!

* * *

Part of not wearing the *daf* on my sleeve (admittedly, I humble-brag about it to my parents and black-hat cousins from Lakewood) has been trying to avoid dressing myself in the weird masculinity and macho of "doing the *daf*." Naturally, I allowed my primary podcast companion to enhance my reading to be "Daf Yomi for Women." Misguided feminism, no doubt. And failed feminism at that, too. In the deeply sexless ether of the anxiety of quarantine, it probably wasn't the best idea to have a woman excitedly learning with me for an hour every day. To be fair, the podcast was as prudish as one could imagine, even as the tractate took us into pretty

---

[2] Jenny Odell, *How To Do Nothing: Resisting the Attention Economy* (New York: Melville House, 2019).

intimate territory: advice about how to lure a lascivious snake out of a vagina with fatty meats and fragrant wines, tongs at the ready to remove and burn it (110a); Rav Chisda's advice to his daughters on foreplay and using modesty to entice suitors (140b); Rabbi Yehuda's report of Rav's claim that Nebuchadnezzar had a 300-cubit-long foreskin when he was trying to rape Zedekiah (149b); and more than 100 mentions of the *zav*, a person who is deemed impure because of his recurrent seminal emissions. I eventually moved from being titillated with anticipation to see how my "Daf Yomi for Women" guide was going to walk us through the dirty bits to being just more eager to hear the squirming and the apologetics for what is by no stretch a feminist book.

In the final analysis, the kind of companionship "doing the *daf*" ended up offering in quarantine was not erotic, but it was romantic, all the same. Not only were my online *havruta* sessions the intellectual highlight of every week, but they also had an emotional punch that was as reliable as it was propelling in a time that motion was hard to generate in all the being still. As quarantine made all time dissolve, the companionship of the page and the people I learned it with helped do the hard work of differentiating the days, marking them up in correspondences and moments of nutty salience. It was a unique form of friendship born of quarantine and Tractate Shabbat: a *nolad*, as it were. It was no wonder that as I cornered the end of the book on 147b, it hit this point directly, drawing from Avot 4:14 (which itself drew from Proverbs 3:5): "If you attempt to quarantine yourself to try to learn, learning won't follow you; you can't rely on your own wisdom, for it is your friends that will cause learning to remain with you." Amen.

* * *

As quarantine eventually eased and I could look forward to the next book, Tractate Eruvin, whose subject would continue to explore boundaries, I knew I would take much from Tractate Shabbat with me, that so many images and passages would return to me as I continue to make sense of the strange new world we are inhabiting. When one finishes one of these books at the *siyyum*, one traditionally says "We will return to you and you will return to us." I noticed the plural this time especially because the most vivid lesson in quarantine was that you have to take your friends with you, in one way or another.

I don't know if I will actually return to Tractate Shabbat in seven-and-a-half years. I certainly know that nothing in the book made me want to become a religious Sabbath observer again or to experiment with trying to keep it wholly or to keep it even a little holy. I didn't leave the book ambivalent about what the actual Sabbath could do for me or my kids in modern times, when we could all use a day without screens.[3] The book barely even tickled my nostalgia bone for the days when my father would read from Abraham Joshua Heschel's meditation on the Sabbath before reciting the blessing over the wine: "In the tempestuous ocean of time and toil there are islands of stillness where man may enter a harbor and reclaim his dignity. The island is the seventh day, the Sabbath."[4] I would erupt in laughter for its pomposity and be sent to my room. Ultimately, my experience with learning about Jewish pausing while on pause myself was singular and without any dissonance, though I'm sure if I do return to the book in seven-and-a-half years again, different pages and passages will make their way into my notebooks.

When the study of the tractate was done (and a new one was starting with significantly fewer restrictions), I came to see *daf yomi*—like the phylacteries Tractate Shabbat discusses on 130 that morph from mere black boxes to white doves, elevating tight straps that bind to a spirituality that helps one soar—as a kind of old-school technology for access to a portal. It provided, and I expect it will continue to provide, like many daily ritual practices, a way to be present and to take oneself to a different plane all at once. To be inside a pause and to have a small opportunity to be outside it in a spiritual and intellectual place with my friends, to be inside and outside of time. As the pages tick off in a regimented way for 2,711 days, reading a book that is some 1,500 years old but still fresh, there is no real day of rest. And I see that that is good: *ki tov.*

---

[3] Judith Shulevitz, *The Sabbath World: Glimpses of a Different Order of Time* (New York: Random House, 2011).

[4] Abraham Joshua Heschel, *The Sabbath: Its Meaning for Modern Man* (New York: Farrar, Straus and Giroux, 1951), 29.

Beezus and Corona: Reading Our
Way Through the Wilderness

Ilana Kurshan

I was fortunate to go into lockdown in a house full of books. Chief among them is the Tanakh I use to chant the Torah portion aloud to my kids each week. We spent the first few months of our lockdown traveling alongside the children of Israel through the desert, to the extent that living through the Coronavirus pandemic began to feel not all that different from traversing "this great and terrible wilderness" (Deuteronomy 1:19). It was in the wilderness that the Israelites were given the commandment to keep Shabbat, and so perhaps it is fitting that I also spent those months reading through tractate Shabbat in the *daf yomi* cycle, learning about desisting from productive labor while so much of life was on hold. It's been hard to get much done with small children underfoot, and like Moses, I've had to contend with complaining and bickering. To distract the kids, I often read aloud to them, hoping that soon they would become readers too. And so I've made my way through this wilderness of a pandemic trailed by an increasingly mixed multitude, including the Israelites, the Talmudic sages, Beezus and Ramona, and the ever-hapless Amelia Bedelia, whose apron has still not worn thin.

There is only one book of the Tanakh that is referred to by name as "in the wilderness," Bemidbar—known in English as the book of Numbers. But the vast majority of the Torah—from the middle of Exodus to the end of Deuteronomy—is set in the wilderness, with its sands stretching endlessly in all directions and no clear landmarks along the way. An entire generation dies out during the forty years of wandering, such that by the time the Israelites enter the Promised Land, no one who had been an adult in Egypt is still alive, with the notable exceptions of Joshua and Caleb. As Avivah Zornberg notes, the wilderness "is not simply a walking surface for the traveling people, but a quicksand ready to consume human bodies."[1] Each morning for the last several months, I have woken up to a message on my phone bearing grim statistics—the number of Covid-19 fatalities,

---

[1] Avivah Gottlieb Zornberg, *Bewilderments: Reflections on the Book of Numbers* (New York: Schocken, 2015), xi.

the number of critically ill patients, the rate of virus transmission. And yet there is something nonsensical about it all—why should a microscopic virus somewhere in Wuhan, China have overturned our world? And why should it take forty years to travel from the Sinai Desert to Israel? If only we—and the Israelites—had known which voices to heed to avoid this terrible predicament.

Unfortunately, the Coronavirus pandemic, like the wilderness experience, has occasioned several crises of leadership. We have spoken ill of our leaders and questioned governmental policies, or the lack thereof. We have tried to stockpile food and supplies, not trusting those who assure us that there will be new manna tomorrow. We have looked back longingly on our lives before this pandemic, wishing we could return to the way it was then – even as we recognize that Egypt was not all that idyllic. The term quarantine comes from the Italian for "forty days," which is reminiscent of the forty years of wandering. We have been enduring this changed reality for longer than forty days now, and hopefully it will be less than forty years—but sometimes it is hard to tell the difference, given that our sense of time has been so acutely disrupted.

* * *

My own sense of time has retained some degree of normalcy thanks to the *daf yomi* cycle, which—like the cycle of weekly Torah portions—marches on as relentlessly as time itself. People often speak about "studying" *daf yomi,* but I rather think that I "read" *daf yomi*; for the last fifteen years, I have started—or at least tried to start—each morning of my day by reading through a page of Talmud. When I come to difficult sections, I generally do not stop to wrestle with the argumentation; I simply read on, jotting down whatever sense I am able to make of the text.

The pandemic set in just when the global *daf yomi* community began Tractate Shabbat, as I gradually realized that people all over the world were being asked to accept upon themselves an extended period of resting, retreating, and staying in. Here in Israel, the Ministry of Health issued increasingly stringent guidelines every few days regarding the extent to which we were permitted to leave our homes and engage socially: No gatherings of over one hundred became no gatherings of over ten which became no *minyanim* (prayer quora) and no unnecessary social interaction with anyone outside one's own family. First the schools were shuttered;

then the restaurants and malls were closed; and then we were told not to leave home unless absolutely necessary. And so it was while increasingly confined to the private domain of my home that I learned the first chapter of Tractate Shabbat, which begins with a discussion of the limits placed on our interactions with people outside.

In the Torah, one of the defining features of Shabbat is the injunction to stay put: "Mark that the Lord has given you Shabbat… Let everyone remain where he is. Let no one leave his place on the seventh day" (Exodus 16:29). One of the thirty-nine labors prohibited on Shabbat is that of carrying an object from one domain to another. As the reality of this pandemic set in, I realized that each time I left my home, I was potentially carrying germs that could infect those around me; and each time I returned home, I was potentially carrying germs that might infect my family. I found myself fearing that I might unwittingly be a carrier, and that no amount of hand-washing or sanitizing would save the people I love or the communities I am a part of from the threat of contagion.

When I began reading the opening pages of Tractate Shabbat, I encountered a series of hypothetical exchanges between a poor man standing outside of a house, and the homeowner inside. May the poor man reach his hand into the house so that the homeowner might place food in his basket? May he take food out of the homeowner's hand? That is, to what extent are we permitted to engage with those around us who might need our help, or who might be able to help us? I have thought about this question often in the past months, as I've tried to reach out to friends in far more difficult situations than my own—single moms isolated at home with young kids, unmarried friends living alone, an octogenarian friend from the pool who is now confined to her assisted living facility. It is more difficult to make contact without contact, but I am learning how to extend my proverbial basket. I wish I could extend a real hand, but the Coronavirus can be transmitted through touch. Perhaps it should not come as a surprise, then, that the hand of a person has a unique halakhic status and is considered a unique domain (3b). The Talmud teaches (Shabbat 14a) that the Sages decreed that hands are ritually impure because they are "preoccupied"—they tend to touch dirty or impure objects. That is, our hands are not ours alone, because they bear the traces of everything in the public domain that we, as private individuals, have touched.

Navigating the risks of Covid-19, like all aspects of germ theory, requires a leap of faith, if not a suspension of disbelief. We cannot see the droplets that may be infecting others when we touch a doorknob or hug a friend or sneeze into our elbows. And yet we are expected to respond with extreme measures. We are asked to desist from most forms of labor, to avoid unnecessary excursions, to spend time only with our families. And so we've stayed home, working by Zoom in button-down shirts and pajama bottoms in a surreal reality in which the second half of Adar was more topsy-turvy than the first. My husband and I speak of the period of our lives before Purim as B.C.E.—Before the Corona Epidemic. My school-age kids fantasize about what they will do "after the Corona"—after this virus at last has passed and they can climb on the monkey bars and share a bag of popcorn with their friends again. And my four-year-old falls asleep every night asking the same question that is on all our minds: "When will Corona end?" I wish I could simply flip ahead to the end of the book and tell her how many pages we have left, but unlike Tractate Shabbat, which takes five months to complete at the pace of *daf yomi*, this pandemic still has no end in sight.

* * *

After two months of lockdown, in late May, the Israeli school system reopened and my children prepared to go back. As they tried on their masks and gloves and stuffed their bags with alcohol gel and sanitizing wipes in preparation for their return, I followed along in the fifth and sixth chapters of Tractate Shabbat, where the rabbis debate what we (and our animals) are permitted to take with us on the Sabbath when we venture forth from the private domain into the public sphere.

My kids, who had been learning at home, had all their schoolbooks and folders to take back with them, and so their bags were far heavier than usual. They were, in that sense, like the camels in the Talmud saddled with a load too heavy for them, which is forbidden, since animals should not be burdened on the day of rest (51b). My son insisted on wearing three levels of protection—a cloth mask, a napkin with rubber bands tied over his ears, and a plastic face shield with his name written in big block letters on masking tape because otherwise he was unidentifiable. Did he really need all this gear? I suppose for him it was like the amulets discussed in the Mishnah, which are believed to protect their wearers from harm. The Mishnah teaches that a person may wear an amulet if its efficacy has been proven or if it was made by an expert. An amulet against epilepsy, the Talmud teaches, may be worn not just by one who has fallen, but also by one who worries that he will fall (61a). So far, thank God, none of us has fallen prey to this illness, but many around us have not been so fortunate.

This pandemic has trained us to stay away from one another. It is difficult, when venturing out for the first time, not to regard everyone we see as a potential threat. The beginning of Tractate Shabbat teaches about Rabbi Shimon bar Bar Yohai and his son, who emerged from a cave where they'd spent twelve years in isolation and proceeded to burn up everything they saw with their eyes, until a divine voice rebuked them with the words, "Have you come out to destroy my world?" (Shabbat 33b). Ultimately, when we do go out, it should be to seek fellowship and act kindly toward those around us. My kids came home from school and could not tell me a thing they learned in their schoolbooks, but they were all so happy to be back with their beloved teachers and friends. Even at two meters apart and with three masks over their faces, they were able to feel the embrace of their school community.

In Judaism our amulets are often our texts, like the tiny scrolls of parchment we hang on our doorposts and kiss each time we exit or enter. But the gesture, too, has supernal power. I kiss my kids each time they leave the house and each time they return, hoping that this amulet, at least, will work its magic.

* * *

Our amulets are not just the texts we read, but the stories we tell ourselves to guard against our deepest fears and anxieties. One afternoon during the second week after the return to school, my kids came home with quite a dramatic story to tell. Before they had even made it to the sink to wash their hands with soap for the requisite two minutes, the story was already pouring out. "*Ima, Ima,* you won't believe it," seven-year-old Liav told me breathlessly.

Her twin sister Tagel took the words right out of her mouth. "There were *ganavim* in school today! Real *ganavim*! And Doron caught them and now they are in *beit keleh!*" Sad to say, that is really how my kids speak—a sort of Ramah Hebrew, with the less commonly-used nouns in Hebrew and all other parts of speech in English.

Liav would not stand for it. "No Tagel, it's my story, be quiet. I'm telling *Ima.*" The problem of who gets to narrate what has been an issue in our family for years, and is particularly acute for the twins, who have many of the same stories to tell.

Liav has always spoken faster and with greater fluency than Tagel, but Tagel is physically stronger and more agile; so generally in these situations, Liav gets the words out first and then Tagel "accidentally" turns a cartwheel and kicks Liav in the face. I tried to avert this catastrophe.

"Girls, whose class did this happen in?"

"Mine, it's my story," said Liav. Tagel stormed off. I let Liav continue, relieved that it hadn't come to blows.

"OK, so there were thieves in school and now they're in jail?" I repeated back entirely in English.

"Yes, you won't believe it," said Liav. I was already skeptical, but their older brother Matan, who was waiting for me to make him lunch, piped in to alert me that "they need a better *shomer* at school. It's very dangerous. Every time Shilon goes inside for a break, *ganavim* can climb right over the fence."

"I'm sure Shilon is an excellent guard," I assured Matan. "You don't need to worry."

"Not true," insisted Liav. "That's what I'm trying to tell you. Today when Doron was going to the bathroom, he saw *ganavim*. They were trying to steal *mahshevim* from the *hadar mahshevim*."

"Thieves were trying to steal computers from the computer room?" I echoed.

"And they weren't wearing masks!" Liav exclaimed indignantly.

This one had me puzzled, but only for a moment. I was picturing bank robbers in comic books. Don't thieves usually wear masks? But now, in Covid times, when everyone is supposed to be wearing a mask, anyone who isn't is immediately suspect.

Liav went on to relate that Doron—a diminutive first grader, the son of a lawyer and a policewoman—went straight to the secretaries and reported what he saw. The secretaries called the police, who arrived with handcuffs and apprehended the *ganavim*, who were now incarcerated in the *beit keleh*.

"Really?" I asked, still somewhat incredulous.

"Oh yes," said Matan. "It's true. I know it's true. They really need another *shomer* to guard the gate when Shilon has to take a break."

By this point, Tagel, overcome by hunger, had emerged from her bedroom and was sitting at the counter eating the salad I had placed before her. When it comes to salad, they each have their own versions of the same basic story: peeled cucumbers, red peppers, yellow peppers—Liav. Peeled cucumbers, tomatoes—Tagel. Unpeeled cucumbers, red peppers, tomatoes, oil, salt—Matan. They crunched their vegetables heartily and continued to elaborate on the incident. All the kids were determined to impress upon me what seemed to them the most critical takeaway. For Liav, it was Doron's heroism when confronted with real-life criminals in his midst. For Matan, it was the security breach. Tagel just wanted to tell the entire story again herself, which she did, with some embellishment. I tried to make sense of it all, not sure how much to believe.

That night, I happened to be texting Doron's mother, the policewoman, about a homework assignment. After we exchanged a few messages, I added a postscript: "Oh, and by the way, you must be so proud of Doron. I heard all about the thieves." She wrote back with a bewildered emoji: "What are you talking about? For real?" And I realized that I had been duped. "If your son is not a policeman, then my daughter is a creative writer," I responded with a smiley face.

"Liav," I said to her the next morning when she was the first to climb into our bed. "I spoke to Doron's *Ima* last night and she hadn't heard anything about the thieves in school. Did that really happen?"

"Well," she said, "like I told you, it was mostly true."

"Mostly true?" I reminded her of the story in *Bemidbar* about the twelve spies who were sent to scout out the land of Canaan while the Israelites were in the wilderness. Ten of them—all but Caleb and Joshua—returned with a terrifying report about the inhabitants of the land: "The country that we traversed and scouted is one that devours its settlers. All the people that we saw in it are men of great size…and we looked like grasshoppers to ourselves, and so we must have looked to them" (Numbers 14:32-33). The Canaanites weren't really giants. The land didn't really swallow up its inhabitants. The Israelites weren't really grasshopper-sized. But they were scared about entering the land, and their fear colored their perspective.

I think for Liav, as for the spies, the dominant emotion was fear. The return to school after Covid-19 was fearsome and fraught. On one of the first days back, the girls reported that the classroom next door to them had been vacated after the class was quarantined—even the tables and chairs had been removed for sanitizing. I imagine it felt haunting each time they passed by. Liav wanted to believe that there was a superhero who would rescue her from danger, even if that superhero was three feet tall and carried a Sponge Bob backpack. Matan wanted to make sure that someone was always standing guard to keep the bad guys out—whether they are germs or unmasked germ-bearing thieves. No wonder their imaginations were so enthralled by tales of stolen computers—they, like the spies, were finding the images with which to articulate their fears.

Should I have reacted to their account with more skepticism? Skepticism, according to a midrash in *Bemidbar Rabbah* (16:6), was the sin of the spies. They refused to believe God, who assured them that the land was good. The midrash compares it to the case of a king who secured for his son a beautiful wife, but whose son insisted on seeing her first because he did not trust his father. I believed Liav's story because her story was true—it was true to the emotions that she and her siblings were experiencing at school. Sometimes unreliable narrators are the most reliable narrators of all, even if the story they are telling us is not the story we think we are hearing. I'm glad that in Liav's account, the thieves were apprehended and order was restored. I could only hope that the story of our own times, too, would have a happy ending.

* * *

I read through the *parsha* (weekly portion), *daf yomi*, and countless kids' books during the pandemic, but I would be remiss if I didn't mention the cookbooks as well. Like so many people out there, we spent much of our Covid-19 quarantine trying out new recipes. Sometimes our baking was inspired by the books I read with the kids, especially the *Beezus and Ramona* series, by Beverly Cleary, which we began reading at the start of the lockdown. Four-year-old Shalvi, who listened but did not always understand, was constantly confusing "Ramona" and "Corona."

One afternoon I read to the kids about how the Quimby parents made their daughters cook dinner after the girls had complained about the previous night's menu. To their own surprise, Beezus and Ramona prepared a successful dinner, though my kids were rather disgusted by their chicken thighs dipped in banana yogurt and seasoned with chili powder. Inspired by the story, my kids insisted that they wanted to make dinner for our family.

"What do you want to make?" I asked, knowing that I would have to be involved.

"Pretzels!" Matan announced, after he caught sight of the empty pretzel jar in our pantry. "We're making pretzels for dinner." The girls nodded in unison.

I opened my mouth to explain that pretzels weren't dinner, but then I thought better of it. We looked up a recipe for soft pretzels, made the dough together, and then I let the kids shape them into twisted pretzel knots before I dipped them in a pot of boiling water and baking soda, which is apparently how they brown. The pretzels went in the oven and everyone had a hearty—if not exactly healthy—dinner.

That night, my husband and I showed the kids a video about the history of the pretzel. In the video, Mr. Rogers visits a pretzel bakery where a young man ties an apron around his waist and teaches Mr. Rogers all about how pretzels are made. We were quite astonished to learn—at least according to Mr. Rogers' source—that pretzels originated in Italy 1500 years ago as prizes given to Christian children for learning their prayers well; the term *pretzel* comes from *pretiola*, Italian for "little rewards." The three empty spaces in the pretzel represent the three parts of the trinity, and the dough is folded over to resemble arms crossed in prayer.

I couldn't believe it. We had been ingesting the catechism for years. "Does that mean we can't eat pretzels in shul?" Liav asked. "I'm not sure we can eat pretzels at all," I responded, recalling the list of activities forbidden at the end of the sixth chapter of Tractate Shabbat because they resemble the "ways of the Amorites" (67a), an idolatrous nation that fought the Israelites in the wilderness. Eating pretzels was not included in the Talmud's list of forbidden idolatrous practices, of course, but even so, the kids and I were in agreement: The next time we made pretzels, we would shape them into rods instead.

* * *

A few weeks after our foray into pretzel baking, the twins surprised me by asking me to make a cake. It was a few days before my birthday, and I had my suspicions: Was this a cake for me or for them, I wondered, thinking of *parshat Shlach Lecha*, which literally means "send for you," a reference to the spies. As Rashi explains (13:2), the spies were "for you," that is, for the children of Israel, who needed confirmation that the land was indeed a good land.

"*Ima*," they told me, "Please make us a plain cake. A cake with nothing on it. We can't tell you why, but we need it. OK?"

"OK," I agreed. "A sheet cake, right?"

My kids looked puzzled. "Not a sheet cake," said Liav. "A bed cake." I made a plain chocolate cake, hoping it would not disappoint.

On the morning of my birthday, they presented me with the cake I had baked for them, decorated with whipped cream, sprinkles, and two marshmallows on one end. "These are the two pillows, yours and Abba's." I asked them why the cake needed pillows, and Liav shrugged her shoulders matter-of-factly. "Because it's a bed cake," she told me. I still wasn't quite sure what she meant. The cake was accompanied by a card—only now, on my forty-second birthday, had I finally merited to receive a handwritten card from my semi-literate children: "To Ymo yor a grate mothor from the cids," they wrote. I knew I was an Ima and sometimes an Ema, but Ymo was a first. They added a line at the bottom of the card that read, "fancyue Ymo for macen a kcece." For a moment I thought I was being called fancy, but then I realized this was just their phonetic rendering of "thank you Ima for making a cake." Under the word "a" I could see there was a crossed-out "the," and I asked Liav about it. "First I wrote thank you for making THE cake, but then I realized you would know that the cake you made was for you, so I changed it to A cake. So it would be a surprise."

Only several days later did I realize that the whole idea for this bed-sheet cake came from *Amelia Bedelia Bakes a Cake,* in which the hapless but well-intentioned housekeeper wins a baking contest after a similar misunderstanding. As an Ymo, I had underestimated my children, assuming they were merely being literal when in fact they were being literary. It was a literary allusion, but it had eluded me. With a lifetime of reading ahead of them, I could only hope it would be the first of many.

* * *

I finished reading aloud the entire *Beezus and Ramona* series during the very same week that we completed the book of Numbers in the Torah reading cycle. When I came to the final paragraph of the last book, Liav pronounced "*Chazak, chazak v'nitchazek*"—the words typically recited upon completing a book of the Bible. It felt appropriate. The Ramona series, like *Bemidbar,* accompanied us through much of the pandemic—as Ramona grew from an exasperating preschooler to a spunky, self-aware fourth-grader, the Israelites made their way through their desert wanderings, her four-plus years of maturation corresponding to their forty.

When conducting a *siyyum*—a ceremony marking the completion of the study of a particular text—it is customary to review the final pages. The last of the eight books in the Ramona series, *Ramona's World,* culminates in Ramona's tenth birthday party. The party is held in a park, like all birthday parties during this pandemic, and rather surprisingly, there is an excessive preoccupation with germs. Ramona's long-time nemesis, Susan, brings an apple to Ramona's party and insists on eating it instead of birthday cake, because "there might be spit on the cake from blowing on the candles."[2]

Ramona is appalled: "I did not spit on my birthday cake," she tells Susan, who remains unconvinced, insisting that her mother told her that blowing out candles is "unsanitary." Ultimately, Susan comes around and tries a little piece of cake, and Ramona feels even more vindicated when Yard Ape—the boy she loves to hate—runs over to sample a piece before licking his "germy fingers" and wiping them on the seat of his "germy pants." The germy cake wins out over the apples, just as Ramona's messiness and peskiness always win out over big-sister Beezus' well-mannered propriety.

The day after we finished the series, the girls and I went back through the previous volumes, turning the pages quickly and stopping to reminisce each time we came to one of the black-and-white illustrations. "Remember when Ramona ate apples in the basement?" Liav asked me, prompted by one of the pictures in the very first book. How could I have forgotten? Ramona had disappeared to the cellar with a box of apples when her sister Beezus was supposed to be watching her, and there she had defiantly taken one bite out of every apple in the box.

I wondered if the apple Susan had brought to the party was a sort of measure-for-measure retribution for Ramona's original sin in the first book. But before I could share my reflection with the girls, they were already onto the next illustration.

We spent quite a while leafing through the paperbacks, pausing each time we came to a picture so as to recall the scene it captured. It reminded me of the last portion in the book of Numbers, *Masei*, which means "journeys." The text reads like a detailed itinerary of the Israelites' wanderings: "They set out from Rameses and encamped at Sukkot. They set out from Sukkot and encamped at Etham, which is on the edge of the wilderness. They set out from Etham and turned toward Pi-Hahiroth...." (Numbers 33:5-7). Rashi asks why the Torah takes pains to record all these stations in the wilderness, offering a midrashic answer:

> This is like a king whose son was sick so he took him to a distant place to heal him. On their way back, his father began

[2] Beverly Clearly, *Ramona's World* (New York: HarperCollins, 2000), 182.

to enumerate all the separate stages of the journey. He told him: Here we slept, here we caught cold, here you had a headache, etc. (Rashi on Numbers 33:1).

The kids and I journeyed through *Ramona* and *Bemidbar* against a backdrop of much sickness, as first the world, then our city, and then our neighborhood were affected by the rampant spread of the Coronavirus. But it was not always as bleak as it sounds.

One of the many stages in the Israelites' itinerary was the journey from Midbar to Matanah. The term *matanah* means "gift" in Hebrew, and the Talmud (Eruvin 54a) explains that this is a reference to Torah—the gift given to the Jewish people in the *midbar,* the wilderness. My experience of this pandemic has been reminiscent of the Israelites' long and tiresome wilderness wanderings, but it has also been filled with surprising gifts, including the gift of time to read together and the gift of witnessing my restless, flighty butterflies metamorphose into very hungry bookworms. I'd like to hope we are heading toward a more promising future. But I also know that with the end of the Torah reading cycle, we move on not to the promised land, but back to Genesis, where the world is created anew. May the unexpected gifts of this pandemic enable us to forge a path to a better future in which we start, once more, in the beginning.

Time in Unprecedented Times

Receiving the Finite Gift of Life Itself

Zohar Atkins

There is no before and after in the Torah.
— *Sifrei Bamidbar* 64:1

Time present and time past
Are both perhaps present in time future,
And time future contained in time past.
If all time is eternally present
All time is unredeemable.
— T.S. Eliot, "Burnt Norton"

Where were you when I laid the foundations of the earth?
— Job 38:4

1.

The arrival of Covid-19 has altered our collective and individual relationship to time and temporality. Or else, it has clarified our fundamental relationship to time and temporality. It has jolted us from our routine and exposed the fragility of our plans on a planetary scale. Life in a pandemic has felt like one long day of awe. It is a holiday in the way that a fast day is a holiday, in the way that Ecclesiastes says, "It is better to go to a house of mourning than to go to a house of feasting" (7:2). It is a holiday in the sense that it alters our relationship to time itself.

What is new about coronavirus is, paradoxically, that it is not new. Plague was a given for our ancestors, who recognized it as a rebuke from God and a call to change. The great surprise for us is that, despite (or even because of) our technological and scientific advances, we are vulnerable to catastrophe. We humans have exerted great mastery of our natural environment, but we are still at Nature's mercy—which is to say, at God's. Coronavirus reminds us not just of the vulnerability we often deny. It reminds us that denial itself makes us vulnerable.

God blessed humanity "to fill the earth and subdue it" (Gen. 1:8), but God also cursed humanity, saying, "By the sweat of your brow you will eat bread, until you return to the ground, for out of it you were taken; for you are dust, and to dust you will return" (Gen. 3:19). The default position of Western modernity, or secular society, is Genesis 1. The sobering backlash we will increasingly receive as a result of hubris is Genesis 3.

Biblical theology presents us with a paradox—explored virtuosically and iconically in Rabbi Joseph B. Soloveitchik's *Lonely Man of Faith*—that still resonates. We are supposed to be *like* God, but we are also to remember that we are *not* God. The former means that we are required to be creators and agents, while the latter means that we are required to be humble about the limits of what we can and should know and do.[1]

When we discover a vaccine, when we use media and technology to limit the spread of the plague, we are acting *like* God. But when we witness the inadequacy of our efforts, the limits of our understanding, the constraints on our political and cultural life, we discover that we are *not* God.

In the past it was easy to accept that we were not God. We knew less about the laws of nature and how to manipulate them. Today, it is both harder and more necessary. The risk in admitting you aren't God is fatalism—accepting things that you can and should change. But this is a cultural risk we need to take, given that our bias is overweighted to emphasize a (false) sense of control.

2.

I do not remember a specific day on which coronavirus arrived. It was already in the world, and in the news, long before I knew anything about it, long before I acknowledged it. Yet even before there was coronavirus, life was fragile and finite. And when coronavirus no longer occupies our global bandwidth there will still be plenty to worry about. "There is nothing new under the sun" (Eccl. 1:9).

As I write these words the pandemic is a present reality, albeit in a "new phase." We still don't know "when it will end," whatever that phrase might mean. We also don't know what its legacy will be on our customs, values, institutions, and worldview when the pandemic is "over."

Did "9/11" end on 9/12? Did Revelation end after God showed Godself at Sinai? Did the Expulsion from Eden end the day after Adam and Eve

---

[1] Joseph B. Soloveitchik, *The Lonely Man of Faith* (New York: Three Leaves Press, 2006).

were shown the door? Has the Destruction of the Temple ended 2,000 years later?

Great events have the quality of dividing time into "before" and "after." Christians mark their calendar B.C. and A.D. For Jews, the calendar begins with Creation, meaning that the first and perhaps great temporal axis is before and after God said, "Let there be light." The Creation story is the bedrock motif of all that is to come. God repeats Creation by saving Noah from the flood, then again by choosing Abraham for a holy mission, and later by taking the Israelites out of Egypt and giving them the Torah. In the messianic future, imagined by prophets like Isaiah, the world will be re-created yet again.

Events are traumas, even when they are positive. They are literally wounds in time. Events make us say, "We will never be the same."

Yet, most of us don't think of Pearl Harbor, the Battle of Gettysburg, or the Treaty of Ghent, for example, every day. We know there will be a time when Covid-19 is no longer news, but a memory; and a time even further when it is no longer—or barely even—a memory, but history.

As time passes, the eventfulness of events fades and discrete events begin to look similar. Even as events unfold, we can't help but interpret them in light of past experience and tradition.

In the Biblical and Midrashic tradition we see this idea in the notion that the same dramas recur. Cain and Abel reappear in the form of Esau and Jacob, Leah and Rachel, Joseph and his Brothers. Traces of the *Akeida* (Binding of Isaac) story can be found in the story of Hannah giving up her only son, Samuel, to become a priest. Jephthah's sacrifice of his daughter offers yet another retelling. The *Mishkan* (Tabernacle) is a forerunner of the *Bayit* (Davidic Temple.)

One reason we turn to stories, myths, and past precedents for guidance is because they have a beginning, middle, and end. Yet life as we experience it does not follow such a neat narrative arc. We can't know what the end will be, both in the sense of "an end of history" and in the sense of the end of our own lives. We also can't consciously remember the moment of our birth, and have to rely on evidence such as birth certificates and the testimony of those who were there to see us enter the world. But even when those people did see our birth, what exactly did they see? Our origins and ends are deeply mysterious. So beginnings, middles, and ends help us domesticate the mystery. A birth date is like the gate outside Eden, guarded by a flaming sword, keeping us from asking about the things we can never know, like the existence of the soul and where it comes from.

We do the same thing with Covid-19: It came from a wet market; no, a lab. A bat; no, a pangolin. It came because of global warming. It came because of the Jews. It came because of globalization. It came because of governmental incompetence and malfeasance. All our explanations—some more plausible than others, some more conspiratorial than others—provide no end to conversation, but do not get at the heart of the matter, which is unknowable. "The highest heavens are for God, but the earth was given to human beings" (Ps.115:16). We are earthlings who can and should know earthly things, but we cannot know that which God alone knows. "God gives power to God's people" (Ps. 29:11). We have *oz*, power, i.e., technological and scientific capacity. But the psalmist does not say that God gave us omniscience.

3.

To reflect on the significance of an event as it is underway is what it means to live in time, to belong to history. There is no Archimedean point outside of history from which we get to judge our moment. We read the story of Noah seeing the dove and imagine him stepping off the ark, but we read and study that story while we ourselves are in the ark. Imagining Noah through hindsight bias we think that he knew everything would be fine all along. *All's well that ends well.* We don't consider that he might have been anxious, that his family might have had many difficult moments huddled together in quarantine.

(We also don't always consider how hard it is to be Noah, building an ark, when everyone else is carrying on as normal. We all want to be Noah, but most of us, statistically, are not. The "preppers" who have invested in ten-year supplies of goods and underground bunkers were probably feeling some vindication when the price of hand sanitizer soared in March of 2020.)

Likewise, we tell the story of Esther as a story of catastrophe averted. Even those of us who undertake the fast of Esther know a miracle is on the other end. But did Esther's people know it at the time?

The Torah suggests the ancients were not as self-assured as we might presume. God reveals Godself to Moses as "the God of your father, the God of Abraham, the God of Isaac, the God of Jacob" (Ex. 3:6). At the precise moment in Moses's own life when his future seemed so uncertain, he is shown a God who visited his ancestors when they, too, were uncertain.

When Jacob flees Esau for his life, he prays, "God of my father Abraham, God of my father Isaac…" (Gen. 32:9). Jacob does not think of himself as a Biblical protagonist. He looks to his ancestors. Jacob does not say, "It will all work out, the book must continue, and Jewish history needs me to survive." He prays.

The example of Moses and Jacob appealing to their own past is a hint that for the Torah, tradition is not about the beginning or the end, but the middle of life. If even the greats do not feel authentic or confident about their place in the world then, paradoxically, we shouldn't feel inauthentic or unconfident about ours, since we are in good company.

4.

How does the meaning of the Torah change when you consider it not as something studied before Creation or at the End of Days, but as something studied in moments of stress and difficulty? Is this one of the possible meanings of the rabbinic dictum, "The Torah was not given to angels of heaven"? (b. Shabbat 88b). The Torah was not given to beings at peace with their reality, but to beings in angst. It is legible and meaningful, appropriate and helpful, only for beings for whom, as Heidegger puts it, "their own being is an issue for them."[2]

The Talmud (b. Ketubot 77b) teaches that we are not allowed to take away the knife from the Angel of Death. In Shabbat 30b, King David tries to defy death by studying Torah all day long (presumably because Death can't take him while studying). But if Torah is given to and for mortals, then King David's use of Torah as a protection *against* death is a misunderstanding. Torah is not an elixir against non-being, but that which enables us to acknowledge and accept it. Read existentially, the Torah scholar's superpower is not immortality, but a greater capacity to "choose life" (Deut. 30:19)—which means, to choose to be a mortal.

In *Being and Time*, Heidegger makes a now classic distinction between fear and anxiety. Fear, he claims, has an object. But anxiety has none. Fear is about what the world can do to me, all the bad things that can happen, what will be if my plans and hopes fail. But anxiety, which is a deeper, more fundamental structure of existence—or, we could say, consciousness—is

---

[2] Martin Heidegger, *Being and Time*, Translated by John Macquarrie and Edward Robinson (New York: Harper & Row, 1962), 12.

about the brute fact that I am mortal; that my life choices are singular, and irreversible; that I have only one life to live and that I must live with myself at each moment until I am no more.

Heidegger reads Tolstoy's *Ivan Ilych* as an example of how social life can't accommodate—and actively represses—the private anguish that each individual person feels when confronted with the prospect of their own death. Ivan Ilych receives visitors who make small talk and fail to appreciate his incommunicable experience. But once, when Ilych was healthy, he was just like them. On Heidegger's read, we are all like Ilych's friends and Ilych at the same time. We are always dying, but initially and for the most part in denial.

To transpose this reading into a Jewish idiom, we are at once in our very selfhood: Job and Job's friends. Job's friends are the part of our self that is socialized, the persona we have come to call our "identity." Job, meanwhile, is the part of ourselves that is constitutionally unreconciled to the world, perennially defiant and troubled no matter what. Viewed psychologically, it hardly matters whether Job is justified.

One of the strange features of a plague is that we can potentially give ourselves and others more permission to be and to present as Job instead of Job's friends.

And yet, so much of the discourse around coronavirus follows the pattern of avoidance Heidegger calls "idle chatter" (*Gerede*) much like the language of Job's friends and Ilych's visitors. We'd still rather talk about politics and policy than about the fundamental mysteries of being alive and of being mortal that the plague presents.

Still, in turning the city and public space itself into a danger zone, at least for a time, the pandemic has offered us the opportunity to visually witness our private anxiety as a shared condition. It has enabled new norms of compassion, connection, and intimacy that are less typical in "healthy" daily life.

The result is that with greater sorrow has also come greater *kedusha* (holiness). Of course, we want things to be mundane, less dramatic, again. But there is also a sense in which we wonder if some of the elevated aspects of pandemic life can be integrated.

Hannah Arendt writes in *Men in Dark Times* of the warmth that pariah peoples experience from huddling closely together as a result of being shut out of public life. Of course, we should not prefer the ghetto to the arena, disenfranchisement to full citizenship and rights; yet Arendt notes that there is a coziness and closeness in such groups not to be found in majority cultures in modern states.[3]

Without idealizing or romanticizing the warmth that is produced precisely in darkness, we should ask what it offers us that we might try to bring back with us into a post-pandemic world.

The Talmud (b. Pesachim 8a) instructs Jews to search for leavened bread the night before Passover with a small torch, not a large one. Why? Because the point is not to *find* the leavened bread, but to *search* for it. The purpose of the light is not to see objects, but to see the darkness—to see the difference a small light can make in a vast darkness.

Torah in an *et tzara* (a time of plague) is likewise a search for what is wrong with ourselves and society, but perhaps by means of a small flame, not a blazing torch. What we get is not clarity so much as luminescence, small miracles, minor consolations.

5.

Living in a time of plague is about living in a time of waiting without expectation, a state of suspense. Even as we wait around for a cure, better testing, and more information, we have to act, we have to live. But this, in fact, is what Jewish life has always been about. Jews wait for a messianic future in which there will be peace and healing for the world, yet are not exempt from acting in the world as it is.

Rabbinic Judaism, I believe, attempts to hold two conflicting truths simultaneously: 1) our situation on earth is not normal; and 2) we must not make that a pretext for engaging in unsustainable and dangerous "emergency politics."

The Sages teach, "Any generation in which the Temple is not built, it is as if it had been destroyed in their times" (y. Yoma 1a). Thus, even in happy, prosperous, and free times, the Talmud instructs us to realize that something is "off" with the state of the world. This is the rabbis' equivalent of today's call: "Don't go back to normal." And yet, every time Jews celebrate a joyous occasion, there is an equally palpable sense that rebuilding is underway.

> Reish Lakish said in the name of Rabbi Yehuda Nesia: "One may not interrupt schoolchildren from studying Torah, even in order to build the Temple" (b. Shabbat 119b).

---

[3] Hannah Arendt, *Men in Dark Times* (Boston: Mariner Books, 1970).

We need to affirm the severity of the plague and listen hard for what it can teach us, but we should also give ourselves permission and encouragement to experience delight and to build—even in a time of constriction. Mourning the state of the world (the loss of the Temple) *and* finding hope and meaning in it as it is (letting children take precedent over rebuilding it) are complementary.

Read more closely, Reish Lakish implies that the path to rebuilding will not be a quick fix, a construction problem, or *technical* challenge, but will be a multi-generational educational and cultural problem—an *adaptive* challenge.

Let us hope for a future of greater health and flourishing for human life on earth, and let us also remember that life is definitionally finite, and that an end to this plague—or even to plague in general—will not absolve us of the difficult task of being human. "It is not on us to finish the work, nor are we free to desist from it" (Pirkei Avot 2:21).

Aging in Place: A Spiritual Fact of Life

Michael Fishbane

"The candle of God is the human soul (*ner Elohim nishmat ha-adam*), to search the innermost recesses of one's being (*le-ḥapes kol ḥadrei baten*) (Proverbs 20:27). And so it happens that, at some moment, we awaken to the Divine gift of consciousness: a sense of awareness that lights up our lives with reflection and responsibility. This is more than waking from a fugue state—a sense that we are endowed with spiritual potential that may be enhanced or diminished in the course of a lifetime.

For Rabbeinu Yona Gerondi (1200-1263), the light of one's soul is such an opportunity for transcendence—God-given, but in our human hands to search out and cultivate. The ruptures and jolts of the everyday may open cracks for this light to appear, because it can jar us from mindless routine. Even the normal anxieties of aging—with their palpable sense of compromise or constriction—can be smothered by busyness and distraction.

For those who, like myself, entered the dimension of Covid-consciousness with as-yet-unrealized projects, or with plans populated by the nearness of family and friends—these days of confinement have imposed a contraction, or *tzimtzum*, of horizons that is hard to ignore. Qualities of expectation have devolved into quantities of endurance. We try to stay in place—even to be placeholders of ourselves—lest we totter in disoriented anxiety. And in addition, we experience ruptures of continuity and space—the kinds of dislocations that Rabbi Nahman of Bratzlav (1772-1810) portrayed as the shattering and amnesia of "place" (our lost sense of how or where things should be), in his story about the breaking of all cognitive and spiritual vessels ("The Mayse of the Ba'al Tefillah"). And so we now wonder: Is it possible that our present situation (and all its delimitations) can offer a prism of spiritual perception—a "concealed light" (an *'or ganuz*)—in the center-space of our soul? Can *tzimtzum* offer opportunities for spiritual growth? If so, we may also ponder: How might we proceed in this strange period, as we age in place—especially those of us for whom aging is no longer a hypothetical or deferred possibility?

Rabbi Moshe Hayyim Luzzatto (1707-1746) once presented an image that has served me as a word of inner guidance in the quest for God and spiritual growth. We awaken, he said, as seekers in a labyrinth, whose path forward constantly diverges without signposts, and within which our perspective is encased by the surrounding walls—so that we cannot view progress or failure from any higher viewpoint. All we have is our desire to go forward toward a hidden, sacred center, which is itself an image of our longing. Certainty is replaced by faith in the power of tradition to orient our soul and focus or guide this quest. On the one hand, our personal sense of spiritual purpose has been shaped by the values and resources of Jewish tradition; whereas, on the other hand, our soul repeatedly reevaluates its progression.

We therefore proceed by engaging "exegetical fragments" that speak to us (often with the voice we impart to it), in the hope that these texts may help comprise a spiritual compass to redirect our gaze (both within and without). Such halting but hopeful readings constitute a significant part of our modern religious situation; and through them we may strive to find prisms of transcendence—given into our cultural hands but also dependent on our personal initiative. I shall follow this interpretative path in the reflections that follow, seeking a spiritual point of focus and purpose. In so doing, I make no broader claim here than an attempt at personal reckoning and integrity. So please consider what follows an exegetical exercise for the sake of my soul. It is offered in spiritual fellowship to those for whom this way of thinking may provide some guidance or psychological resonance.

* * *

I would like to begin my meditation with a teaching by Rabbi Mordechai Yosef Leiner of Izhbitze (1801-1854), the "Izhbitzer." It is found in the first collection of his sermons, known as *Mei Shiloah*, and takes up the verse, "Abraham became old (*zaqen*), entering the [fullness of] days (*ba' ba-yamim*); and the Lord blessed Abraham with *kol* ("all" or "everything")" (Genesis 24:1). Immediately after this citation, the Izhbitzer first cites another Scriptural text; and then, after a series of clarifications, sets forth his own theological insights:

> It is written "And this is my portion (*helqi*) from all (*mi-kol*) of my labor" (Ecclesiastes 2:10). This verse occurs in the *Gemara* (Sanhedrin 20b) and is explicated there by both "Rav and Samuel: the one (Rav) explained the word *helqi* to mean *maqli* ("my staff"); whereas the other (Samuel) said it meant *qodi* ("my

vessel"). Thus [we learn] that King Solomon (the speaker of these words) trusted in God and did not complain, heaven forbid, about the loss of pleasure (his portion) in this world, since he did not consider it of value; but proudly states that though it seemed he was deprived of everything (*kol*), the gist "of all" (*mi-kol*) his years remained, and with this he would make the most of life. [This comment explicates the citation.] "This is my portion of all my labor"—for the person (Rav) who explained "my portion" as "his staff" considered this latter to be an allusion to "life"; namely, the "strength of life" remaining to him, as Scripture states: "A person with his stave in his hand [from the totality of his days]" (Zechariah 8: 4). And the person (Samuel) who explained the word "portion" to mean "his vessel" deemed this an allusion to a "receptacle" (*keli qibbul*) ready and yearning for an addition. This latter (the "addition") refers to his (Solomon's) enjoyments—for this was the essence of life in this world. All this [explains] the [meaning] of the verse, "Abraham became old, entering the [fullness of] days"—[that is,] he entered the sources of [true] life, and was a vessel to receive and desire the surplus [bounty] of life from God—ever more on each occasion.[1]

The foregoing passage, despite its cryptic and elusive formulations, offers two orientations toward temporality and life experience—one centered on King Solomon, who is the subject of the quotation from the Book of Ecclesiastes (traditionally attributed to him); the other on Abraham, who is the subject of the Torah verse cited at the outset (Genesis 24:1). R. Mordechai Yosef Leiner cites the two passages in tandem, ostensibly because the adverb *kol* occurs in both. But he begins his exposition by adducing two explanations of the word *helqi* ("my lot" or "portion") from the Talmud (the one by Rav, who said it meant *maqli*; the other by Samuel, who said it meant *qodi*), because the context there dealt with a series of verses from Ecclesiastes where Solomon had attained certain things (notably, the accumulation of wealth) "earlier" in his reign, but was left with little "at the end" (in this case, only his staff).

The Izhbitzer uses this loss of material gain to state that Solomon disregarded this factor with consummate trust in God, and focused instead

---

[1] *Sefer Mei Shiloah* (Vienna: A. Della Torre, 1860), 9b.

on the life that remained (the years left "of all" his allotted number). Thus the image of the staff (the marker of what remained of his gain) was reinterpreted to symbolize the strength and determination he had to make the most of his final years (the citation from Zechariah 8:4 is adduced to reinforce that interpretation). From an image of loss it was transfigured into a positive image of reliance on God. Similarly, the image of a vessel is used to speak of Solomon's desire to draw forth enjoyments from the well of life in the days left to him. He thus exemplifies a path of purpose, making the most of his remaining life.[2]

If Solomon is a paragon of religious trust—marking individuals who, despite material losses, use their religious and psychological strength to attain the fullness of final days, Abraham is a paradigm for a different theological ideal. His distinctive trait in old age is to "enter the days" of his life with spiritual focus and vigor—to turn to the Source of life, to God, and to become like a receptive vessel, or *keli qibbul*, that yearns for the increase of the gifts of Divine "Life." His central concern was not to focus on the quantity of mortal days left to him but to seek their spiritual quality: entering time as a spiritual dimension of transcendence of Divine beneficence in the everyday.

This is a theological orientation that desires to exceed the quantified temporalities of our normal, ordinary life (as Rabbi Levi Yitzhak of Berditchev noted, in a discussion of this verse in his *Qedushat Levi*),[3] and turn to the realm of eternal life—to the sphere of Divinity. This spiritual stance does not disregard or deny the elements of God-given life during one's lifetime; but focuses on the illuminations that are revealed within the particulars of daily existence—a radiance that connects us to a time-transcending eternity. How so?

Let us think further about the models of our two religious personalities.

The spiritual concern of Solomon was to recognize the limitations of time, and to seize life-moments with determination and psychological strength. But this is a stance that turns time into space—that quantifies lived reality into a series of slots, some filled and others left vacant, and looks to the

---

[2] It is notable that the Izhbitzer's quote from the Talmud uses the word qod (vessel), rather than gondo (cloak), which occurs in the traditional Vilna edition—probably on the strength of Rashi's use of the variant qod, adduced by Rav Hai in his remarks on Toharot, Mishnah Kelim 16.1. This reading was accepted by Rabbi Yoel Sirkis, the Ba"H, and is confirmed by the Munich manuscript of the Talmud.

[3] See *Sefer Qedushat Levi Ha-Shalem*, edited by M. Derbaremdiger (Brooklyn, NY: Machon Qedushat Levi, 1991), I, 54-55.

future as occasions to fill gaps of experience. Time is here but an occasion for acquisitions, suggesting that whatever one has done is insufficient and must be filled by activities at the next available moment. Having strength and accumulating experience is thus essential for such an orientation; even as one is repeatedly assessing whether a particular or anticipated task is the right one—whether it measures up to expectations. For such a person, time and life are viewed as extensions and things to be added up, as if the vessel one uses to gather experiences is a measuring cup.

But the vortex of life-crises and an unending lack of fulfillment undermine this perspective. If we need a pandemic or simply aging to impel a different orientation, so be it; but certainly all the anxieties of quantification have been chipping away at our resistances all along. Hence, for all its "basic trust" in the God-given world as a sphere for achievements, the model of Solomon has practical limits—for it can devolve into mere busyness. For that reason (and more), the stance of Abraham as formulated by the Izhbitzer may help reposition the axes of our spiritual life. For based on this reorientation to time, we may "enter the days" of our lives in and through their immediate presence, in the course of our engagement with what is happening as it happens. So lived, time has a qualitative dimension given to us by our readiness to be present to it. This is an act of *tzimtzum*, or contraction of consciousness, that is transformative. It is a stripping away of the deleterious psychological sense of a "not-yet" expectancy—an attitude that fills time with both tension and anxiety (this being an adult version of the "fear of missing out").

Thus, "aging with Abraham" is aging into the sacred mystery of ever-present eternal life, since it transcends the undertow of a presumptive something still-to-come—something that will always be still-not-this. How, then, can one become a *keli qibbul*, or "receptive vessel" for the *now* that is always already here and now? How can we overcome the desire to be out and about (and not confined), or the fear of living an incomplete or unrealized life?

Since I have been emphasizing the qualities of time over their quantification, how can this concern be conjoined to the mysteries of place? Can time and space be converging spiritual vectors?

* * *

Space is locative. This is more than an apparent redundancy; it is a fact of our concrete experience. We are either here or there, moving between places, in full cognizance of these movements and transitions; or in a mindless trance, being creatures of habit. Sometimes we anticipate a new location and move toward it in both mind and body; at other times, we find ourselves suddenly in a place that is unexpectedly holy or profane, and our heartbeat and body register this experience. Furthermore, we carry an interior space within us as memories—and because of this, there is a palpable feeling of unease between our inner spaces (vibrating in older time warps) and the outer places where we are standing. These are some of the features of a phenomenology of space that affect our seeing something from afar or from within, or the sensations that pulsate and evoke muscle memory.

Crossing a threshold has its own tonalities, and going in or out is never neutral. Home is evocative and equivocal, since its enclosures may be alternatively protective (both in fact and in recollection) or constraining. And truth be told, this dual modality has come to the psychic surface for many of us during these "at-home" days of the pandemic. Brooding about these matters has reevoked for me the memory of reading, many decades ago, Gaston Bachelard's *The Poetics of Space*. It seemed then, as it does now in retrospect, to have an oracular quality, and set my inner compass of reflections about spatiality—and especially what it means to be grounded. I learned to think then, for the first time, about the shifts in mental movement and the immensities of motionless quietude, while daydreaming around a silent center.

This gaze inward seeks God-abounding, when we open our inner eye. And precisely this sensibility was perceived by the ancient sages when they pondered the meaning of Scripture which said that Tamar sat at a place called *Petah Einayim* (Genesis 38:14). For where, they wondered, was this site located—so otherwise unknown? Not letting this problem of outer geography deter them, we are told that this location refers to the place of inner yearning—*petah einayim* being the locus toward which one's spiritual eye is opened; the place of spiritual longing toward which we are spiritually oriented (Genesis Rabbah 85.7). Our true place is where our inner eye opens to seek beyond. The pilgrimage of the heart is the pang of spiritual pathos.

These thoughts have returned to me repeatedly during these days, as I have pondered the qualities of inner space. In an uncanny way, one of the first times of confinement following the outbreak of the virus was when the Scriptural portion of the week was *Be-Shalah*—a reading that reports the giving of manna from heaven: to be gathered during the weekdays only; not on the Sabbath when the injunction was *al yetzei ish mi-miqomo*—when each person was enjoined "not to leave their home." The word *miqomo* (literally, "place") in the law alternates with the word *ohel* ("tent") in the narrative (Exodus 16:15, 29), and served even more poignantly to underscore the stay-at-home regulations then pronounced by the authorities.

The *tehum Shabbat* of later rabbinic rulings (this marking the fixed outer boundary of travel on the Sabbath day) is hereby contracted to one's home—and even more, according to many Hasidic masters, to one's inner space, to the settled interiors of spiritual consciousness. The turmoil of daily labor, of gathering what is needed for sustenance and survival, has its psychic correlate in the felt sense of restlessness or appropriation—the need to fill the gaps of want through endless acts of distraction; whereas the repose of the Sabbath, when physical procurements are prohibited and we must rely on what has been collected, has the spiritual correlate of contraction, through the inward quality of rest.

During the time of gathering, there is a constant process of "going out" with some quantitative purpose—each person determining what is functionally needed or possible. According to a perceptive midrashic gloss on the diverse sensibilities of taste (*ta'am*) that characterized the manna, we are told that each individual construed its quality and "meaning" according to their age and "ability"—since it was palpably different for the young or elderly, and satisfied their bodies and minds accordingly (*Pesiqta de-Rav Kahana* 16. 25). This is not a throwaway exegetical figure (evoked by the dual sense of the word *ta'am*, as both "taste" and "meaning"), but rather hints at a confusion of perception when one's thoughts are mired in the mindset of material acquisitions or external needs.

For the daily gatherers, the mysterious substance that so pervaded the earth evoked the question "*Man hu*, what is it?—because they didn't know what it was, [asking] *mah hu*" (Exodus 16:15). Not knowing, each person thus answered or responded according to their "ability" (*koah*), as the Midrash put it. That is, they reduced the question of mystery to a definable "thing" or substance, referencing or correlating it to what was previously known to them, and in their own terms. They were unable to direct the question inward or ask, as did Moses prior to this episode, when he countered the complaints of the people (against himself and Aaron), with the words, *ve-anahnu mah* (Exodus 16:7). Thinking from a spiritual orientation or perspective, later teachers transformed this remark from a query asserting mortal inability ("*Mah*, who are we"—that you complain against us?!) into the striking existential assertion: "We are *mah*!" Doing so, they acknowledged their mortal finitude and allowed the puzzlement of quiddity (the *whatness* of things) to enter the very core of their being—ideally, they proclaimed, even an act of self-nullification into the ineffable "Nothing" (or *ayin*) of Divine reality (notes the *Qedushat Levi*).

Hence living with a *mah*-consciousness required a maximum act of divestment and receptive rest, one that allows the state of not-knowing to pervade one's inner being. Perhaps this is also what Rabbi Ephraim Lunshitz (1550-1619), the *Keli Yaqar*, perceived when he evoked the rabbinic adage that the revelation of Sinai was only given to *okhlei ha-man* ("those who ate the manna")—and reinterpreted it to refer to those who could internalize this deep state of spiritual receptivity, and thereby transform a mode of inquiry (of *man?*, meaning "what?") into a quality of lived existence.

* * *

Let me return to my original theme, and the question that underlies this foray through the sources (a personal collection and evaluation of texts). Is it possible to age in place—that is, to live in a manner other than with quantified expectations; to accept the challenge of Abraham's openness to the unfolding of presence? And if so, how might we formulate this? I offer the following possibility as a speculative gesture.

Our primary "place" is the prism of spiritual perception in our soul, and the correlations repeatedly effectuated between it and all the mysteries of the external world. Our sense of "being *mah*," as a fundamental configuration of consciousness, may then find its exterior coordinate with experiences of the world that evoke the question of primary wonder: *Man hu?* This disposition must be cultivated; for if a sense of *thingness* comes to our awareness from moment to moment, ever neutral in nature, we can transform it by an act of open receptivity. Conjoining one's inner (existential) sense of *mah* to the omnipresent potential of events to evoke awe and reverence (epitomized by the evocation *Man hu?!*) is more than an epistemological correlation. It is, I would suggest, a theological bonding, or *devequt*, with God's unbidden giving and manifest creation, received with reverent wonderment. It is a cleaving of the mind to the sacred God-given vitality of existence, to the wondrous sustenance that fills the universe.

Thinking along these same lines, one of the first disciples of the Ba'al Shem Tov, Rabbi Uri Fievel (c. 1739-1806), the "Maggid of Dubienka," in his work *Or He-Hokhmah*, suggested that the *man* (manna) is an ontological reality or transcendental manifestation of all the bounties materialized in our world. In his view, to appreciate and experience this, our consciousness must divest itself of all externality, and perceive the inner light of God's omnipresent creativity as a sacred radiance within reality. Or, in the terms that I have been using, the spiritual task is to strive to connect (with a receptive intentionality) to the givenness of reality as expressions of the Divine bounty of things. And when we come to this awareness, we may also perceive that the external world conceals the query of *man?* or *mah?*—this evocation being the depth dimension of our perceptions *and* the spiritual focus of our consciousness. To raise the question *man hu?* is to give our attention to the inestimable unknowns pervading existence and allow the spiritual qualities thereby evoked to radiate into the spaces of awareness.

This spiritual posture is significantly different from the quantifications of the life-world mentioned earlier, and allows our sense of being housed in a body to be qualitatively transformed. This is, I may add, a spiritual state that is experientially "beyond time"—not in the metaphysical sense so often discussed in Hasidic sources (most notably in the *Sefas Emes*, by Rabbi Yehudah Aryeh Leib of Gur, 1847-1905), but in the theological sense of being at a crossing point between eternity and temporality. At this nexus we are at the still point of awareness, and the world is present with God-given revelations. On these occasions we may even sense God's transcendent truth shining on our souls, opening our hearts to the sacred question— *Man hu?* Beyond self-consciousness, and all our manipulative calculations, things just are: *mah nora ha-maqom ha-zeh,* "how awesome is this place!" Not knowing how it happens, or when, we are addressed in life, in a sacred *now*—beyond the discontinuities of time. We then may "enter the days" of our lives as into eternity: daily "gradations" of expanded awareness, a God-consciousness beyond all knowing (*Zohar* 1. 129b).

Ner Elohim nishmat ha-adam

le-ḥapes

Author Biographies

Deena Aranoff is Faculty Director of the Richard S. Dinner Center for Jewish Studies at the Graduate Theological Union in Berkeley. She teaches rabbinic literature, medieval patterns of Jewish thought, and the broader question of continuity and change in Jewish history. Her recent publications engage with the subject of childcare, maternity, and the making of Jewish culture.

Zohar Atkins is the Founder and Director of Etz Hasadeh and the author of *Nineveh* (Carcanet Press, 2019) and *Unframing Existence* (Palgrave Macmillan, 2018). A Rhodes Scholar and a poet, he writes a weekly Torah commentary newsletter at etzhasadeh.substack.com.

Rachel Sabath Beit-Halachmi is an American-Israeli rabbinic leader, author, and public speaker. She is the incoming inaugural Senior Rabbi of Har Sinai-Oheb Shalom Congregation in Baltimore, MD. Most recently, Dr. Sabath served as Assistant Professor of Jewish Thought and Ethics and led a four-campus team at the Hebrew Union College-Jewish Institute of Religion (HUC). For 25 years, Dr. Sabath has taught courses on modern Jewish thought, ethics, liturgy, theology, gender, and Zionism. Currently she serves as a senior fellow at the Kaplan Center for Jewish Peoplehood. She is presently at work on two volumes, one on the dilemmas of modern Jewish thought, and the other, co-edited with Rachel Adler, a volume on ethics and gender in Judaism. Among Rabbi Sabath's published works are *Preparing Your Heart for the High Holy Days* and *Striving Toward Virtue*, both of which she is a co-author.

Michael Fishbane is the Nathan Cummings Distinguished Service Professor of Jewish Studies at the University of Chicago. He has written many articles and scholarly books that span Biblical and Midrashic literature, Medieval Bible Commentaries, and Hasidic thought. His theological works include *Sacred Attunement: A Jewish Theology*, and the forthcoming *Fragile Finitude: A Jewish Hermeneutical Theology* (University of Chicago Press, 2021). Fishbane is a Fellow of the American Academy of Jewish Research and the American Academy of Arts and Sciences.

Arthur Green was the founding dean and is currently rector of the Rabbinical School and Irving Brudnick Professor of Jewish Philosophy and Religion at Hebrew College. He is also Professor Emeritus at Brandeis University. Both a historian of Jewish religion and a theologian, his work seeks to form a bridge between these two distinct fields of endeavor. He is the leading figure of Neo-Hasidism in the contemporary Jewish world, seeking to articulate a contemporary Jewish mysticism based on the Hasidic model. His most recent writings include the two-volume *A New Hasidism*, co-edited with Dr. Ariel Mayse (JPS, 2019), a translation of the Hasidic classic *The Light of the Eyes* by R. Menachem Nachum of Chernobyl (Stanford, 2020), and *Judaism for the World: Reflections on God, Life, and Love* (Yale, 2020).

James Jacobson-Maisels is the founder and executive director of Or HaLev: Center for Jewish Spirituality and Meditation (http://orhalev.org). He was the founding Rosh Yeshiva of Romemu Yeshiva and has taught Jewish thought, mysticism, spiritual practices, and meditation at the Pardes Institute of Jewish Studies, Haifa University, Yeshivat Hadar, and in various settings around the world. He received his PhD from the University of Chicago.

David Zvi Kalman is Scholar in Residence and Director of New Media at the Shalom Hartman Institute of North America. He leads the Kogod Research Center's research team on Judaism and the Natural World. David Zvi received his PhD from the University of Pennsylvania. His research touches on Jewish law, the history of technology, technology and ethics, material culture, and Islamic jurisprudence. He is the owner of Print-O-Craft Press.

Ilana Kurshan is the author of *If All the Seas Were Ink*, published by St. Martin's Press and winner of the Sami Rohr Prize for Jewish Literature. She has translated books of Jewish interest by Ruth Calderon, Benjamin Lau, Yemima Mizrahi, and Micah Goodman, and she is a regular contributor to *Lilith Magazine*, where she is the Book Reviews Editor. Kurshan is a graduate of Harvard University (BA, summa cum laude, History of Science) and Cambridge University (M.Phil, English literature), and she teaches at the Conservative Yeshiva in Jerusalem, where she lives with her family.

Sara Labaton is the Director of Teaching and Learning at the Shalom Hartman Institute of North America. She has a PhD in medieval Jewish thought from NYU's Skirball Department of Hebrew and Judaic Studies and has taught in various Jewish educational settings.

Yitz Landes is a PhD candidate in Religion at Princeton. His research focuses on the reception history of rabbinic literature and Jewish liturgy. His first book, *Studies in the Development of Birkat ha-Avodah*, was published by the Mandel Institute of Jewish Studies in 2018.

Ethan J. Leib is the John D. Calamari Distinguished Professor of Law at Fordham Law School. He is the author or editor of five books—the most recent two about loyalty and friendship—and teaches courses about contract law and legislation.

Jon A. Levisohn is the Jack, Joseph, and Morton Mandel Associate Professor of Jewish Educational Thought at Brandeis University, where he also directs the Jack, Joseph, and Morton Mandel Center for Studies in Jewish Education.

Ayelet Hoffmann Libson is a scholar of Talmud and Jewish law and is an associate professor of law at the Interdisciplinary Center, Herzliya. In 2017-2018 she was the Gruss Visiting Professor of Jewish Law at Harvard Law School. She teaches courses on rabbinic literature, the history of Jewish law, and the intersection between religion and human rights. Her publications have appeared in journals such as the *American Journal of Legal History, Oxford Journal of Law and Religion, AJS Review,* and *Jewish Quarterly Review.* She is the author of *Law and Self-Knowledge in the Talmud* (Cambridge University Press, 2018).

Ariel Evan Mayse joined the faculty of Stanford University in 2017 as an assistant professor in the Department of Religious Studies and serves as the rabbi-in-residence at *Atiq: Jewish Maker Institute* (atiqmakers.org). Previously he was the Director of Jewish Studies and Visiting Assistant Professor of Modern Jewish Thought at Hebrew College in Newton, Massachusetts. Mayse holds a PhD in Jewish Studies from Harvard University and rabbinic ordination from Beit Midrash Har'el in Israel. He is the author of *Speaking Infinities: God and Language in the Teachings of the Maggid of Mezritsh* (University of Pennsylvania Press), and co-editor of the two-volume *A New Hasidism: Roots and Branches* (Jewish Publication Society, 2019). He is working on a forthcoming monograph examining the relationship between spirituality and law from the dawn of Hasidism to the eve of the twentieth century.

Shaul Magid is Professor of Jewish Studies at Dartmouth, Kogod Senior Research Fellow at the Shalom Hartman Institute of North America, and rabbi of the Fire Island Synagogue. His forthcoming book, *Meir Kahane: An American Jewish Radical,* will appear with Princeton University Press.

Aviva Richman is Rosh Yeshiva and faculty member at Hadar Institute in Manhattan. Her doctorate from New York University is in Hebrew and Judaic Studies, with a dissertation on sexual consent and coercion in the Babylonian Talmud. Richman is a graduate of the Wexner Graduate

Fellowship and also a graduate of the Center for Jewish Law at Cardozo Graduate Fellowship in Jewish texts and legal theory. She received private ordination following a traditional course of study in Jewish law, from Rabbi Elisha Ancelovits and Rabbi Danny Landes in Jerusalem.

Devorah Schoenfeld teaches Judaism at Loyola University Chicago. She received her PhD from the Graduate Theological Union in 2007 and received ordination from Yeshivat Maharat in 2019. She has written on Jewish-Christian relations, medieval biblical interpretation, and comparative theology. Her previous book, *Isaac on Jewish and Christian Altars* (Fordham University Press, 2012), compares Jewish and Christian medieval interpretations of Isaac's near-sacrifice. She is currently working on a book on the theological implications of the *Song of Songs* in medieval exegesis.

Chaim Seidler-Feller is Director Emeritus of the Yitzhak Rabin Hillel Center for Jewish Life at UCLA, after 40 years of serving students and faculty. Chaim received Rabbinic ordination from Yeshiva University, where he completed a Masters in Rabbinic Literature. Chaim has been a lecturer in the Departments of Sociology and Near Eastern Languages and Cultures at UCLA and in the Department of Theological Studies at Loyola Marymount University. He is also a faculty member of the Shalom Hartman Institute of North America and the Wexner Heritage Foundation. He was the founding director of the Hartman Fellowship for Campus Professionals and a founding member of Americans for Peace Now.

Erin Leib Smokler is Director of Spiritual Development and Dean of Students at Yeshivat Maharat Rabbinical School, where she teaches Hasidism and Pastoral Theology. She is also a Research Fellow at the Shalom Hartman Institute of North America. She earned both her PhD and MA from the University of Chicago's Committee on Social Thought, and her BA from Harvard University. She was ordained by Yeshivat Maharat. Leib Smokler previously served as Assistant Literary Editor of the *New Republic*, and her writing has appeared there, as well as in other publications. She is currently at work on a book entitled *Torah of the Night: Pastoral Insights from the Weekly Portion.*

Joshua Teplitsky is an associate professor in the Department of History and the Program in Judaic Studies at Stony Brook University. He specializes in the history of the Jews in Europe in the early modern period. His current work explores public health, Jewish life, and epidemics. He earned his PhD from New York University's Departments of History and Hebrew & Judaic Studies and has held fellowships at the Oxford Center for Hebrew and

Jewish Studies of the University of Oxford, the Katz Center for Advanced Judaic Studies at the University of Pennsylvania, the National Library of Israel, and Harvard University. His first book, *Prince of the Press: How One Collector Built History's Most Enduring and Remarkable Jewish Library* (Yale, 2019), was a finalist for the National Jewish Book Award.

Gordon Tucker is Vice Chancellor for Religious Life and Engagement at The Jewish Theological Seminary of America (JTSA). He is also currently a Senior Fellow at the Shalom Hartman Institute of North America. Having served as Senior Rabbi at Temple Israel Center in White Plains, NY, from 1994 to 2018, he is now Senior Rabbi Emeritus. He holds the A.B. degree from Harvard College, a Ph.D. from Princeton University, and Rabbinic Ordination from JTSA. From 1984 to 1992 he was the Dean of the JTSA Rabbinical School. He is the author of scores of articles on Jewish theology and law, and published *Heavenly Torah*, a translation of, and commentary on, Abraham Joshua Heschel's three-volume work on rabbinic theology. Most recently, his new commentary on *Pirkei Avot* was published by The Rabbinical Assembly in 2018.

Tamara Mann Tweel is Director of Civic Initiatives at the Teagle Foundation. Previously, she served as the Director of Strategic Development for Hillel International's Office of Innovation, where she founded and directed Civic Spirit, a multi-faith civic education initiative. She currently teaches in the American Studies Program at Columbia University, the Shalom Hartman Institute of North America, and serves on the Advisory Council of The Princeton University Office of Religious Life. Dr. Tweel received a master's degree in theological studies from the Harvard Divinity School and a doctorate in history from Columbia University. Her work has been published in numerous academic and popular journals, magazines, and newspapers, including *The Washington Post, The Harvard Divinity Bulletin, The Journal of World History* and *Inside Higher Ed.*